# PSYCHIATRIC DRUGS FOR THE NON-MEDICAL MENTAL HEALTH WORKER

*By*

## WILLIAM GOLDSMITH, M.D.

*Staff Psychiatrist*
*Brentwood Veterans Administration Hospital*
*Los Angeles, California*
*Assistant Clinical Professor of Psychiatry*
*University of California at Los Angeles*

*Illustrated by*

## Linda Ellen Leib

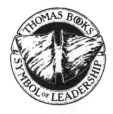

CHARLES C THOMAS • PUBLISHER
*Springfield • Illinois • U.S.A.*

*Published and Distributed Throughout the World by*
**CHARLES  C  THOMAS  •  PUBLISHER**
Bannerstone House
301-327 East Lawrence Avenue, Springfield, Illinois, U.S.A.

© *1977, by* **CHARLES  C  THOMAS  •  PUBLISHER**

ISBN 0-398-03635-7

Library of Congress Catalog Card Number: 76-54198

*With* THOMAS BOOKS *careful attention is given to all details of
manufacturing and design. It is the Publisher's desire to present books
that are satisfactory as to their physical qualities and artistic
possibilities and appropriate for their particular use.* THOMAS
BOOKS *will be true to those laws of quality that assure a good name
and good will.*

*Printed in the United States of America*
*R-2*

*Library of Congress Cataloging in Publication Data*

Goldsmith, William, 1938-
    Psychiatric drugs for the nonmedical mental health
worker.

    Includes index.
    1. Psychopharmacology.   I. Title
RC483.G63        615'.78        76-54198
ISBN 0-398-03635-7

to Joel
Class of '00

# INTRODUCTION

THIS book is based on the belief that non-medical mental health workers should learn about psychiatric drugs.

The field of psychopharmacology — the study of drugs which affect the mind — has advanced immeasurably in the past twenty years. Countless numbers of drugs have become available for the relief of anxiety, depression, the psychoses, and behavior disorders. More and more is becoming known about the drugs themselves. However, many patients are wholly or partially under the care of therapists who have had no formal medical training: psychologists; psychiatric social workers; pastoral and lay counselors; occupational, recreational, and music therapists; and various paraprofessionals.

With the burgeoning of the community mental health movement and the successful drug treatment of the chronic psychoses, thousands of former mental hospital patients now receive services at outpatient clinics, day-treatment centers, board-and-care-homes, and halfway houses. Most of these patients take psychotropic drugs, but have little contact with physicians and nurses. Their day-to-day contact is mainly with non-medical mental health workers.

Since medication is a major part of the treatment of so many of their clients, non-medical practitioners should have some background in the area of psychopharmacology. They should know when and what kind of a drug may be indicated, its expected effects, and its possible side effects. They should be prepared to refer a patient for

medication, and to monitor drugs' actions between con-
tacts with the prescribing physician. This is not to say
they should be expected to prescribe medication or regulate dosage. However, their observations may be crucial to
the doctor who makes these decisions.

Many mental health workers are in conflict about psychotropic drugs. They may oppose their usage, employing
such phrases as "chemical straightjacket," "making zom-
bies out of patients," or "doping them up." Sometimes
there is truth to these assertions; patients may be improp-
erly medicated. Such feelings are often partly due to mis-
conceptions about the drugs themselves.

Other practitioners, while not antidrug, may feel anxious and helpless when a patient complains about his
medication. Is the patient's complaint realistic or a manifestation of his emotional disorder? Should the therapist
overstep his bounds and discourage continuation of the
drug? Is the drug addicting? Suppose the patient overdoses? There is probably no experienced clinician who has
not been tortured by these and other drug-related ques-
tions.

This text is intended to give the non-medical mental
health worker a basic understanding, in some depth, of
psychotropic medication. To achieve this, some knowledge of human anatomy and physiology is essential. Part I
is intended to fill the latter need. Part II is devoted to the
drugs themselves.

The attempt has been made not to burden the reader
with unnecessary terms and concepts. Those which are
presented are essential. To be useful, this text cannot be
read casually. Except as noted, mastery of the material in
Part I and its correlation with Part II is advised. To this
end, there is extensive cross-referencing. Some readers may
find it helpful to consult pertinent bibliographic refer-
ences.

Those mental health workers who remain "antidrug"

may find support for their position here. There is no minimizing of the potential hazards of drug therapy, nor of the limitations of the drugs currently in use. It is hoped, however, that the receptive clinician and student will gain information and concepts which will enhance his effectiveness in serving his patients. The aim of this text is better patient care.

W. G.

# CONTENTS

# PSYCHIATRIC DRUGS
# FOR THE NON-MEDICAL
# MENTAL HEALTH WORKER

# Part I
# Drugs and the Body

# CHAPTER 1

# THE ADMINISTRATION OF DRUGS

$H$OW are drugs taken? This may seem to be a simple question, with an obvious answer — "pills and shots." But what about drugs applied to the skin, intravenous medications, or inhaled drugs? A detailed discussion of drug administration provides an illuminating review of practical anatomy and offers an important perspective on psychopharmacology. In a systematic way, from the surface of the body inwards, the administration of drugs will be surveyed.

## Skin

The skin is composed of several layers which vary in thickness over the body: The skin on the inner surface of the wrist is thin; on the back it is thick. The basic layers are the *epidermis*, composed of rapidly reproducing cells functioning as a protective barrier between the body and its environment; the *dermis*, in which hair roots, sweat glands and sensory nerve endings are situated; and the *subcutaneous* area, where fat provides insulation and smaller blood vessels channel into capillaries (see Fig. 1).

A medication may be applied directly to the skin, either to treat a dermatological condition or to be absorbed into the system. An example of the former is calamine lotion applied to an itchy rash; an example of the latter, a liniment whose purpose is to warm and stimulate underlying muscles. (Most preparations of this type only stimulate superficial blood flow, causing a pleasing, but placebo warmth.)

A drug may be administered by injection into any layer of the skin. A needle might stop in the epidermal or

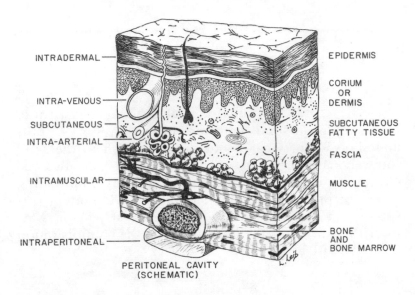

INTRADERMAL — EPIDERMIS

INTRA-VENOUS — CORIUM OR DERMIS

SUBCUTANEOUS — SUBCUTANEOUS FATTY TISSUE

INTRA-ARTERIAL — FASCIA

INTRAMUSCULAR — MUSCLE

INTRAPERITONEAL — BONE AND BONE MARROW

PERITONEAL CAVITY (SCHEMATIC)

VARIOUS SITES OF INJECTION

Figure 1.

dermal layer; a drug injected there is termed an *intra-dermal injection.* An example is a tuberculin skin test. It is injected intradermally so that the body's reaction, usually a red, raised area, can be visually observed, and so that very little of the drug will be absorbed into the general circulation.

A needle might stop under the dermis, a *subcutaneous injection,* an example of which is a tetanus-toxoid injection. This site permits slow absorption and is useful for the administration of substances which might be irritating if injected into the next major tissue area muscle.

## Muscle Injections

Most drug injections, psychotropic or otherwise, are

given intramuscularly. The muscles of the shoulder or buttock area are the usual sites of injection because of their mass. Drugs injected into muscle are absorbed rather quickly, because most muscles are richly vascularized. The drug quickly enters the general circulation and usually reaches higher concentration than when given orally. However, when giving an intramuscular (I.M.) injection, care must be taken that the needle has not entered a blood vessel. Many drugs given safely I.M. would be dangerous if injected directly into the circulation.

### Intravenous and Intraarterial Injections

The most direct method of administering a drug is via the circulatory system. A drug may be injected into a vein or, much less commonly, an artery. Drugs given in this manner are carried to all parts of the body in a matter of seconds, in contrast to the minutes to hours of intramuscular injection. Also, the drug reaches body organs without having been affected by digestive processes, or liver and/or muscle enzymes (see p. 24).

### Intraperitoneal, Intrathecal and Bone Marrow Injections

Still following the path of the needle, and for the sake of completeness, these uncommon, but possible, routes of drug administration will be mentioned. A drug may be injected directly into the abdominal cavity, where it will be rapidly absorbed. This is termed an *intraperitoneal* route. A needle inserted into the area surrounding the spinal column is in the *intrathecal* space. Spinal anesthesia is administered here. Conceivably, but very rarely, a needle might be inserted into the marrow cavity of the bone. Drugs given here will also be rapidly absorbed.

## The Intestinal Tract

Any mucosal surface may absorb a drug. This means
that the absorption of a drug into the body may begin in
the mouth itself. Nitroglycerine, a medication used in
some cardiac conditions, is given in tablets which are
placed under the tongue. The tablets dissolve in the saliva
and are absorbed directly into the circulation through the
mucous surface under the tongue, into the plexus of veins
in this area. *Sublingual* administration, as it is termed, is a
fast way to administer highly soluble drugs.

Traveling down the esophagus or food tube, the drug
reaches the stomach. There is relatively little absorption
into the general circulation from the stomach itself. The
tissues of the stomach are adapted for storage and digestion, rather than absorption. Depending on such factors as
the amount and type of food in the stomach, and the age
and general health of the patient, it takes one-half to one
hour for drugs in the stomach to move into the upper
small intestine, where most absorption occurs (see Fig. 2).
This is of clinical importance. It means that drugs taken
orally have a comparatively slow onset of effect, but because of the rate of absorption, a relatively long period of
action. In cases of overdoses, evacuating the stomach
within one-half to one hour may prevent toxic effects.

It should also be pointed out that the digestive tract has
two ends. Drugs can also be administered rectally. Drugs
administered in suppository form are well absorbed. His-
torically, before intravenous administration was available,
fluids were given to unconscious patients via the rectum.

## Inhalation

Absorption of drugs in the respiratory tract may begin
in the nose, which is lined with an absorbent mucous
membrane. Heroin, morphine, cocaine and snuff are examples of drugs so administered.

The lungs provide an immense area of tissue through

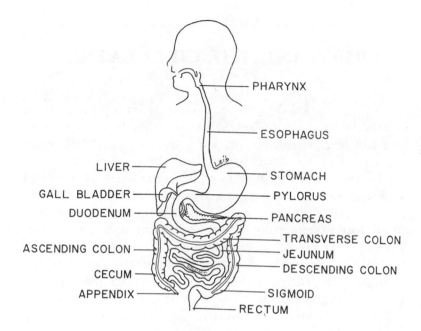

PHARYNX

ESOPHAGUS

LIVER

STOMACH

GALL BLADDER

PYLORUS

DUODENUM

PANCREAS

TRANSVERSE COLON

ASCENDING COLON

JEJUNUM

DESCENDING COLON

CECUM

APPENDIX

SIGMOID

RECTUM

ILEUM - WHERE THE MOST DRUG ABSORPTION OCCURS.

## DIGESTIVE SYSTEM

Figure 2.

which absorption of biologically active substances may occur. Anesthetic gases are drugs administered through the lungs. The advantage of this route is that it is fast, and the duration of administration can be well controlled. Smoking may be considered as a way of administering nicotine via the respiratory tract.

### Other Routes

It is theoretically possible to administer medication through the mucosa of the vagina, the conjunctivae (linings of the eyes) and the lining of the urethra.

# CHAPTER 2

# DRUGS AND THE CIRCULATION

THE previous chapter is essentially an outline of how drugs get from the outside environment into the body's circulation. This section deals with what happens after the drug passes into the circulation.

The circulatory system may be considered as a closed track; beginning at any point, it is possible to trace a return to the starting place. In considering drug distribution, the circulatory system may be broken down into several elements: *blood circulation, lymphatic circulation* and *cerebrospinal fluid* (CSF). In order to delineate these systems without going into detailed anatomy, the possible route of a dose of oral medication will be traced (see Fig. 3).

The drug is absorbed into the blood through a capillary in the wall of the upper small intestine. From this microscopically tiny blood vessel, it passes into progressively larger vessels until it reaches a small vein, which drains blood from the gut wall. It may then pass into a larger vein called the *portal vein*. This takes it to the liver, where the drug may be acted on by a multitude of enzymes (see p. 24).

At this point, the drug may be destroyed by enzymatic action or passed from the liver into the bile, the digestive secretion of the liver. Bile is secreted by the gall bladder into the upper small intestine. Here the drug may be reabsorbed again and passed back into a capillary.

Some drugs become trapped in a circuit known as the *entero-hepatic circulation*, passing from the gut to the liver and back again. It should be emphasized, however, that the drug may pass through the liver without being excreted, and stay in the general circulation before being

10

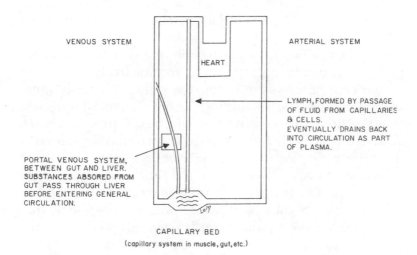

VENOUS SYSTEM

ARTERIAL SYSTEM

HEART

LYMPH, FORMED BY PASSAGE
OF FLUID FROM CAPILLARIES
& CELLS.
EVENTUALLY DRAINS BACK
INTO CIRCULATION AS PART
OF PLASMA.

PORTAL VENOUS SYSTEM,
BETWEEN GUT AND LIVER.
SUBSTANCES ABSORED FROM
GUT PASS THROUGH LIVER
BEFORE ENTERING GENERAL
CIRCULATION.

CAPILLARY BED
(capillary system in muscle, gut, etc.)

SIMPLE SCHEMATIC OF CIRCULATORY "TREE"
SHOWING ARTERIAL, VENOUS & LYMPHATIC SYSTEMS

Figure 3.

caught in the entero-hepatic circulation again.

Assuming the drug passes unchanged through the liver or instead gets into a vein which bypasses the liver altogether, it may then enter the largest vein in the body, the *inferior vena cava*. This vein empties into the right side of the heart, a chamber called the *right atrium*. From the right atrium, the blood passes through a valve into a thick-walled chamber, the *right ventricle*. It then passes into a large vessel, the *pulmonary artery,* which branches into smaller and smaller vessels which eventually become the capillaries of the lungs. It is here that blood gets rid of $CO_2$ and is reoxygenated.

Going through progressively larger vessels, the drug passes back to the *pulmonary vein* and into the *left atrium* of the heart. From the left atrium, it goes into the *left ventricle* and out into the general circulation through the largest artery, the *aorta*. It then may pass into any part of the arterial tree, from head to toe, to any tissue. It may then pass out of the capillary system and into the fluid which surrounds most cells.

Capillary walls, being only one or two cells thick, are permeable, permitting substances to pass freely in and out of the capillaries surrounding the cells. Cell membranes may also act to pull substances from the circulation out into the fluid surrounding the capillary, a process known as active transport. From the fluid surrounding the cells, the drug may pass into the *lymphatic system.*

Lymph is essentially plasma, the fluid which carries the blood cells. The lymphatic system plays a relatively minor role, so far as is known, in psychopharmacological action. It is sufficient to say that lymph eventually returns to the arterial system.

Moving to another part of the arterial tree, the drug may be carried into the area of the brain itself. Carrying the drug to the capillaries of the brain does not insure that the drug will get into the brain. While oxygen and smaller molecules diffuse easily enough from capillary to brain tissue, the brain is relatively impervious to many larger molecules, including most drugs. This physiological circumstance is called the *blood-brain barrier.* Essentially, this means that it is difficult for most drugs to penetrate the brain. The concentration of drug in the brain may be only a tiny fraction of its concentration in the blood, or in other body tissues. Of course, some drugs must penetrate the blood-brain barrier, or no psychoactive drug would have any effect at all. In clinical practice, this means that a large amount of most drugs must be present in the rest of the body, for a small amount to permeate the brain. This is one of the main reasons many psychoactive substances must be taken in such large quantities that they cause undesirable side effects.

The brain is bathed and cushioned by a liquid, *cerebrospinal* fluid, which circulates around the brain and down the spinal column. A lumbar puncture permits the taking of a sample, and studying it is important in evaluating various neurological diseases. Metabolic products of drugs can be recovered from the CSF. It is also possible to administer drugs via the CSF, such as spinal anesthetics and antibiotics.

The actual circulation of a drug through the circulatory system takes much less time than it does to tell about it. Depending on the heart rate, the timespan may be less than thirty seconds for a drug molecule to pass from the gut, through the body and back to its point of entry. The same applies to a drug absorbed from its site of injection in a muscle, introduced directly into a vein by intravenous drip, inhaled through an anesthetic mask or rubbed on the skin.

## Plasma Binding

After a drug enters the circulation, several things may happen to it before it exerts any action.

When a drug passes the capillary wall, it is in the general circulation. It has entered the medium of blood. Blood is composed of cellular components and plasma. The cellular components are red blood cells, which conduct oxygen via hemoglobin, and the much less numerous white blood cells. There are various types of white cells. Some of their functions have a bearing on drug action; this will be discussed in later sections. As with any other tissue, the blood cells themselves may take up drugs.

The drug may stay in the plasma, the fluid component of the blood. Plasma is composed of water, enzymes, various salts and chemicals, and a class of compounds called proteins. These are large organic molecules which have various complex functions. With respect to drug action, it is important to note that the drug molecule may become attached, or *bound*, to plasma proteins.

When a drug is bound to a plasma protein, its pharmacological action may be reduced or completely eliminated. When bound to a plasma protein, the drug cannot easily pass out of the circulation to its site of action or other tissue. The part of the molecule which activates the target tissue receptor may be covered by the plasma protein. The activity of a drug is inversely related to its degree of binding to plasma proteins (Fig. 4).

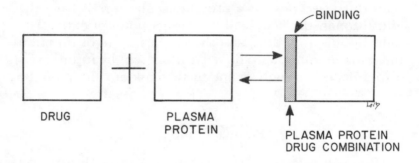

DRUG     PLASMA PROTEIN     PLASMA PROTEIN DRUG COMBINATION

BINDING

**PLASMA PROTEIN BINDING OF DRUGS**

Figure 4.

## Distribution and Selective Accumulation

From the discussion of circulation and the blood-brain barrier, the point arises that drugs do not go only to the area for which they are intended. An antibiotic given for a throat infection also penetrates other parts of the body, where no physiological need exists.

Some drugs have a tendency to accumulate in certain tissues. It is well known that DDT amasses in fatty tissue. Iodine tends to accumulate in the thyroid gland; lead concentrates in bone.

Some drugs must be taken until there is an adequate

general tissue saturation before their maximum desired effect is obtained. Digitalis, a medication which increases the strength of cardiac contractions and influences heart rhythm, is such a drug. A patient must take it in large doses for the first few days before changing to a smaller or *maintenance* dose.

## Drug Elimination

In subsequent sections, the mechanisms of metabolism of the absorbed drug will be described. This section deals with how a drug is eliminated from the body, whether or not metabolism has taken place.

Drugs, as is the case with anything else taken into the circulation, may be excreted back into the external environment. The most common routes of excretion are, of course, through the urine and feces. Drugs may also be eliminated through the skin, hair, tears, saliva, maternal milk, lungs, nails, and teeth.

The fate of an administered drug will be examined with respect to its excretion. Some of the drug may not be absorbed at all into the capillaries of the G.I. tract. If the medication is taken with food, it may pass through the intestinal tract and be eliminated in the feces without ever having exerted any biological effect. For this reason, many drugs are given between meals and/or at bedtime in order to minimize mixture with food.

Some of the ingredients in food itself may interfere with the absorption of the drug. Tetracycline, a common antibiotic, if given with milk or milk products, reacts with the calcium in the food, forming an insoluble compound which cannot be absorbed.

Usually, some of the drug is absorbed. As mentioned above, it may pass to the liver and be excreted in the bile. This is the mode of excretion of many drugs. The drug itself, or its metabolic products, is then eliminated in the feces.

Other drugs are not excreted by the liver. Eventually, during their passage in the circulation, they pass through

# MOUTH

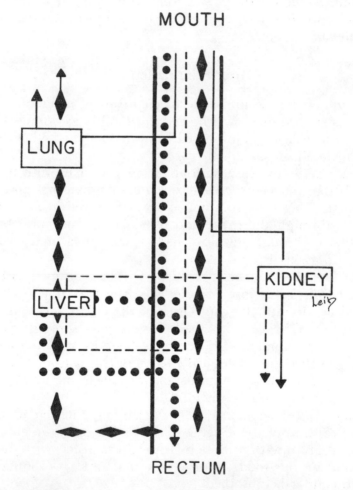

# POSSIBLE ROUTES OF EXCRETION
# OF AN ORALLY ADMINISTERED DRUG

Figure 5.

the *renal arteries,* the vessels which supply the kidneys. These drugs pass out of the renal circulation and into structures called *glomeruli.* These are specialized cellular organs which may be very roughly compared to filters. Drugs or their metabolites pass into the glomular filtrate and into the urine, which is excreted through the bladder and urethra (see Fig. 5).

Some drugs are eliminated by both the liver and the kidney, and others, by one only. A drug's principal mode of excretion is sometimes of clinical importance. For example, if a patient has impaired kidney or liver function due to disease, doses of medication should be reduced. Lower dosage will still result in adequate concentration of the drug because excretion has been impaired. An overdose of a drug which is excreted by the kidneys may be treated with renal dialysis.

# CHAPTER 3

# DRUG METABOLISM

W HEN a drug enters the body, it enters an environment in which literally millions of chemical reactions are occurring continuously. The body has apparatus for dealing with foreign substances so they will either support and maintain body function or be rendered inert and harmless. Food, for example, may be considered a foreign substance which is subjected to digestion in order to fuel the body's physiology, maintain tissues, and promote growth and healing.

Drugs may be considered a specialized type of food, and are subjected to the same processes. A drug often will not perform its pharmacological action in the same form in which it was ingested. It must be chemically changed, *metabolized*, before it becomes pharmacologically active.

On the other hand, metabolism of many drugs renders them physiologically inert. The study of the metabolism of drugs is important in understanding their action and also may lead to the development of new drugs. Some drugs on the market are only a metabolic transformation of another drug. These are often advertised as being faster-acting drugs. From a commercial standpoint, it means that the patent on the older drug can be avoided, and an almost identical medication can be sold under a different name.

The mechanisms of metabolism will be discussed under the section on enzymes. This section will briefly describe some basic metabolic processes. The details of these processes are not especially important in clinical practice. They are presented to give increased scope and appreciation of the process of drug metabolism and to introduce terms that occur in drug literature.

## Oxidation

Oxidation is the combination of a compound with oxygen. It also means loss of electrons at the atomic level. The presence of oxygen is not necessary for oxidation to occur. The result of oxidizing a compound is the release of energy, which may be used by the system, and the breakdown of the compound into smaller molecules, which may then be excreted more easily.

In the body, many simple organic compounds, including some drugs, are broken down into carbon dioxide ($CO_2$), water ($H_2O$) and urea ($NH_2$-C-$NH_2$) by oxidation. This process affects mainly compounds with a "straight chain" of carbon atoms, called *aliphatics*.

## Reduction

Reduction refers to gain of electrons at the atomic level. In terms of body chemistry, it generally means the addition of hydrogen. This process is sometimes responsible for the production of active metabolites from a relatively inactive drug.

## Conjugation

Some substances are soluble in a fatty, or *lipid*, medium. Others are only soluble in a watery, or *aqueous*, medium. Whether a drug, or food, is water- or lipid-soluble is often of great importance. A substance may have to be lipid-soluble in order to pass through the gut wall and water-soluble in order to be excreted in the urine.

Conjugation is the metabolic process which attaches one compound to another, often changing its solubility. An important example occurs in the liver, where a compound called glucuronic acid conjugates with bilirubin, a lipid-soluble breakdown product of hemoglobin. Hemoglobin is the oxygen-carrying molecule present in red blood cells.

Since about three million red blood cells are created and destroyed every second, the body must have some mechanism of excreting the red cell hemoglobin released by this process. It is first broken down to bilirubin. As the bilirubin passes through the liver, it is conjugated to glucuronic acid, forming a water-soluble compound which is then excreted through the bile system and into the gut, where it is further broken down by bacterial action. Feces are colored brown because of this mechanism of excretion of old hemoglobin.

When a patient is jaundiced, it may be due to a blockage in the biliary system of excretion of conjugated bilirubin. The bilirubin "backs up" into the bloodstream, eventually coloring the skin yellow. In addition, other types of conjugation occur, some of it with drugs.

### Exchange

A compound may lose one atom and simultaneously gain another, becoming a different compound. An example of this is the exchange of a sulphur atom for an oxygen atom in the conversion of the barbiturate thiopental to pentobarbital (see Chapter 17).

### Excretion Unchanged

There are drugs, for example, some inhalation anesthetics, which pass through the system unmetabolized and are structurally unchanged.

### Other Aspects of Metabolism

Most drug metabolism occurs in the liver, a seething hotbed of enzymes; some occurs in the kidneys, and probably all tissues are capable of some drug metabolism.

Metabolism may be altered by the general state of the system. Infants, for example, do not have a well-developed ability to metabolize drugs. The elderly often have reduced liver and kidney function and metabolize medications more slowly. This is one reason that drug dosages are reduced at the extremes of age. During illness, a medication may be metabolized more rapidly, as the body temperature is higher, increasing the rate of the chemical reactions involved. Aspirin is metabolized more rapidly during rheumatic fever.

The presence of certain drugs, such as barbiturates, stimulates the metabolism of other drugs, a process called *induction*. Induction refers to the increased activity of some enzymes which act on drugs.

The body's ability to metabolize a certain drug may increase as the drug is administered. There is probably an increased production of the enzymes necessary to metabolize the drug. Therefore, an increasing amount of the same drug may be required in order to achieve the same pharmacological effect. This is one of the mechanisms (but only one) involved in the phenomenon of *tolerance* to drugs, or *drug dependence* (see p. 75). For example, a patient who is addicted to barbiturates may be able to take very large amounts without much effect, achieving blood levels which would be fatal to a non-addict. This is partly due to the body's development of an increased ability to metabolize barbiturates.

# CHAPTER 4

# ENZYMES

THE chapter on metabolism dealt with what happens to a drug in the body. How it happens is the subject of this chapter.

Basic chemistry teaches that the speed of chemical reactions is influenced by the temperature at which the reaction takes place. When a test tube containing a solution is held over a Bunsen burner, a color change or the bubbling up of a gas may occur, visual manifestations of some chemical transformation.

In the body, however, the temperature is, and must be, relatively stable. Bunsen burner heat would curdle the proteins which make up much of animal tissue. Since millions of chemical reactions are happening all the time in the body, other influences must be at work.

A *catalyst* is defined as a substance which influences the speed of a reaction, without participating in, or being changed by the reaction. Enzymes are catalysts. They cause the myriad reactions which occur in the system.

An *enzyme* is an organic chemical substance produced by a living organism which modifies the speed of a reaction. It is neither used up nor does it appear as a reaction product. Enzymes are proteins. All of the reactions described in the section on metabolism are enzyme-mediated. An understanding of basic enzyme theory is essential to the understanding of the action of some psychotropic drugs.

It is not known how many enzymes are present in the normal body. Only a relatively few are well defined, and only a few are so well known that familiarity with them is essential to an understanding of psychopharmacology. However, this number is likely to increase steadily.

Much about an enzyme may be learned from its name.
The name is derived from the substrate on which it acts by
adding *ase*. For example, the class of enzymes which split
fat are *lipases*. The enzyme which metabolizes acetyl cho-
line is called *acetyl cholinesterase*.

Enzymes are produced by genes. One gene produces one
enzyme. Genes are located in chromosomes in the nuclei of
cells. Enzymes, therefore, are produced intracellularly.
They concentrate in the cytoplasm of cells, in structures
collectively called the *endoplasmic reticulum*. This submicroscopic apparatus consists largely of structures called
*microsomes, ribosomes,* and *mitochondria,* which are anatomically adapted as sites for enzyme action (see Fig. 6).

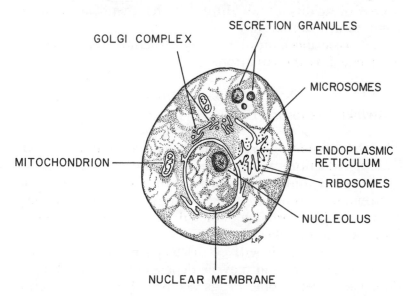

**STRUCTURE OF A CELL
SHOWING ENDOPLASMIC RETICULM**

Figure 6.

There are also free-floating enzymes which are present in the general circulation and in other areas of the body. The liver is the most enzyme-rich organ. As discussed above, all materials absorbed from the gut may pass through the liver, to be acted upon by the enzymes present in the liver tissue. Most drugs are metabolized by *hepatic (liver) microsomal enzymes.*

Enzyme action itself is affected by several factors. The gene which produces the enzyme may be stimulated or repressed by environmental factors controlling the concentration of the enzyme. The concentration of the substrate on which the enzyme acts, and the products of the enzyme-catalysed reaction set up an equilibrium. The pH, the degree of acidity or alkalinity of the chemical environment, is also important.

The basic mechanism of enzyme action, then, may be represented as the equation:

$$E + S \rightleftharpoons E\text{-}S \longrightarrow \text{Products of Reaction} + E$$
$$\text{(enzyme)} \quad \text{(substrate)}$$

The above equation represents the enzyme activity in oxidation, reduction, and synthesis. An enzyme may act to split a compound. It may carry a hydrogen atom from one compound to another. It may conjugate (join) two compounds or build smaller molecules into large proteins to form muscle or other tissue.

Drug action, as it will be discussed in detail, is influenced by enzymes and may be dependent on them for action. Conversely, some drugs act by influencing specific enzymes.

In clinical medicine, measurement of enzyme activity is often of diagnostic importance. For example, if a patient suffers a *myocardial infarction* (heart attack), there is damage to heart tissue. The damaged cardiac cells release enzymes into the general circulation. Some enzymes, while also occurring elsewhere in the body, are highly concentrated in cardiac tissue. The enzyme level can be measured in the serum and, if elevated, indicates damage to the heart. Measurement of enzyme level also provides some indication of the healing process, as the level will decrease as the cardiac injury heals.

Similarly, liver enzymes will be elevated in cases of hepatitis or other liver disease. An elevated level of Serum Glucose Oxaloacetic Transaminase (SGOT), may be indicative of liver or heart damage.

The enzyme *monoamine oxidase* (MAO) catalyzes oxidation of compounds with one amine (NH2) as part of their structure. Since many neurotransmitters are monoamines, this enzyme is important in psychopharmacology. A class of antidepressant drugs acts by inhibiting the action of MAO, thus causing a buildup of those compounds whose metabolism is dependent on MAO.

CHAPTER 5

# THE PERIPHERAL
# NERVOUS SYSTEM

IT is paradoxical that relatively little is known about what psychiatric drugs actually do in the psyche. There are many theories, but knowledge is limited in understanding how psychotropic drugs work in the brain. There is detailed information, however, about how these drugs act in other parts of the nervous system. The nervous system, other than the brain and spinal cord, is known as the *peripheral nervous system*. It is important for the non-medical practitioner to have some acquaintance with its anatomy and physiology. Complaints about side effects are often due to the action of psychotropic drugs in the peripheral nervous system.

## Spinal Cord and Voluntary Nerves

The lower portion of the brain extends into the long column of nervous tissue, the *spinal cord*. The spinal cord contains tracts of tissue which carry neural impulses from the brain to the body and from the body to the brain. Nerves arise from the spinal cord and go to various areas. They are *spinal nerves,* and contain fibers which carry impulses between the brain and the muscles. The spinal nerves innervate muscles which are under voluntary control, such as those of the hands, arms and legs.

## The Autonomic Nervous System (See Fig. 7)

In addition to the nerves which direct voluntary motor

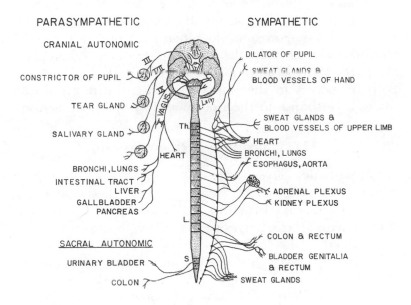

PARASYMPATHETIC    SYMPATHETIC

CRANIAL AUTONOMIC

DILATOR OF PUPIL

CONSTRICTOR OF PUPIL

SWEAT GLANDS &
BLOOD VESSELS OF HAND

TEAR GLAND

SALIVARY GLAND

SWEAT GLANDS &
BLOOD VESSELS OF UPPER LIMB

HEART

BRONCHI, LUNGS

ESOPHAGUS, AORTA

BRONCHI, LUNGS
INTESTINAL TRACT
LIVER
GALLBLADDER
PANCREAS

ADRENAL PLEXUS
KIDNEY PLEXUS

COLON & RECTUM

SACRAL AUTONOMIC

URINARY BLADDER

BLADDER GENITALIA
& RECTUM

COLON

SWEAT GLANDS

SCHEME OF THE AUTONOMIC NERVOUS SYSTEM

Figure 7.

activity, there is another set which connects the brain with internal organs, such as the heart, lungs, liver, and kidneys. It connects with muscles which are not generally under voluntary control, such as the muscles in the wall of the intestines.

There are connections with the glands which regulate body physiology, the *endocrine system* (see Chapter 8). These nerves further innervate sweat glands, the tiny muscles of hair roots, and areas lined with mucous membrane, such as the lining of the nose and the mouth. Of great importance is their innervation of the *circulatory system* — the heart and blood vessels. Collectively, this set of nerves is called the *autonomic nervous system.*

The system of autonomic nerves is subdivided into two types called *sympathetic* and *parasympathetic nerves.* Most autonomically innervated structures are served by both types of nerves. They generally exert opposite or contrasting effects. For example, when the pupil of the eye is stimulated by its sympathetic nerves, it dilates. When parasympathetically stimulated, it contracts. If the parasympathetic nerves to the pupil were cut, the pupil would dilate in response to the unopposed sympathetic action.

## The Sympathetic Nervous System

Sympathetic nerves originate from a portion of the spinal cord which is in the area of the chest and lower back, an area called the *thoraco-lumbar system*. Stimulation of sympathetic nerves causes physiological responses, as outlined in Table I.

When any nerve is stimulated, an impulse travels to the end of the nerve, the *synapse*. A synapse is defined as the anatomical relation of a nerve cell, or *neuron*, to another cell. The synapse may be with another neuron, a receptor on a gland or a muscle cell. The area between the nerve ending and the tissue innervated is the *synaptic cleft* (see Fig. 8).

When the nerve impulse reaches the synaptic cleft, a chemical substance is released. It crosses the synaptic cleft to the receptor, causing stimulation of the receptor. Depending on where the receptor is located, stimulation may result in muscle contraction, release of a hormone from a gland or stimulation of another neuron. The substance which stimulated the receptor is then either destroyed by enzyme action (see Chapter 4) or taken back up into the nerve cell. If the nerve cell is stimulated again, the substance may be rereleased.

These substances are *neurotransmitters*. Their release, destruction, and reuptake is almost instantaneous. This mechanism permits precise regulation of the duration of neuronal activity.

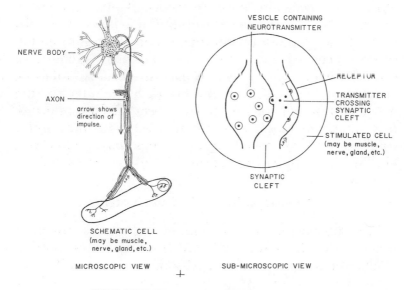

NERVE BODY —

AXON

arrow shows
direction of
impulse.

SCHEMATIC CELL
(may be muscle,
nerve, gland, etc.)

MICROSCOPIC VIEW

VESICLE CONTAINING
NEUROTRANSMITTER

RECEPTOR

TRANSMITTER
CROSSING
SYNAPTIC
CLEFT

STIMULATED CELL
(may be muscle,
nerve, gland, etc.)

SYNAPTIC
CLEFT

SUB-MICROSCOPIC VIEW

NERVE SYNAPSES AND THE SYNAPTIC CLEFT

Figure 8.

In the sympathetic portion of the autonomic nervous system, the principal neurotransmitter is called *noradrenaline* or *norepinephrine*. Sympathetic activity is sometimes called *adrenergic transmission*. Another neurotransmitter released by some sympathetic nerves is *epinephrine,* which has a chemical structure very similar to noradrenaline.

The tissue receptors which are activated by adrenergic transmission are called *adrenergic receptors*. They are divided into two main groups; *alpha-* and *beta*-adrenergic receptors. Noradrenaline only stimulates alpha-receptors. Epinephrine stimulates both alpha- and beta-receptors. Many organs and tissues have both alpha- and beta-receptors.

In the circulatory system, alpha-stimulation by norepinephrine results in constriction, or narrowing of blood vessels. Beta-stimulation by epinephrine causes dilatation, or widening of vessels. Muscle in vessel walls has both alpha- and beta-adrenergic receptors. Alpha-stimulation contracts the muscle; beta-stimulation relaxes it. In the heart, beta-receptors predominate, and their stimulation causes increased heart rate and increased strength of cardiac contractions. If there is excessive beta-stimulation, an oversensitivity of heart muscle with irregular rhythm may result (see Chapter 9). In fact, there is a class of drugs, *beta-adrenergic blockers,* which are used in various cardiac conditions. Some psychotropic drugs have adrenergic blocking or stimulating action, as will be discussed.

### Parasympathetic Nervous System

This subdivision of the autonomic nervous system arises from part of the brain itself, and from the lowest portion of the spinal cord. For this reason, it is also called the *cranio-sacral system.* As is the case with the sympathetic system, there is parasympathetic innervation of internal organs, including the heart, lungs, salivary glands, intestinal tract, and the genito-urinary system. Parasympathetic stimulation results in the physiologic responses outlined in Table I.

A state of mild, generalized parasympathetic stimulation usually occurs after a satisfying meal. It is a time of rest and recuperation, a physiologic state promoting conservation of energy and rebuilding of tissue. In contrast, the sympathetic system may be thought of as mediating the "fight or flight" response, preparing the system for emergency action. To shift the analogy, the sympathetic system is the body's accelerator; the parasympathetic system is the brakes. Both systems are in a constant state of activity, and ideally, they act in balance. If one is excessively stimulated or blocked, a state of physiologic imbalance results.

The principal neurotransmitter of the parasympathetic system is called *acetylcholine.* Stimulation of parasympathetic nerves results in the release of acetylcholine into

Table I

Effects of Stimulation of the Sympathetic and
Parasympathetic Nervous System

| Organ | *Sympathetic Stimulation* | *Parasympathetic Stimulation* |
|---|---|---|
| Eye | Dilated pupil tearing | Contraction of pupil, |
| Heart and Blood Vessels | Increase in heart rate, higher blood pressure, increased blood volume, constriction (narrowing) of most blood vessels | Slowing of the heart, dilatation of blood vessels supplying the intestinal tract |
| Lungs | Relaxation and widening of bronchi (air tubes of the lungs) | Constriction (narrowing) of bronchi |
| Digestive System | Thick viscid saliva, decreased gastric secretion, slowing of the intestinal tract, increased release of sugar from storage in liver | Increased watery saliva: Increased peristalsis (gut motion); stimulation of gastric secretions |
| Urinary and Reproductive Organs | Relaxation of bladder, constriction of sphincter muscle of bladder (greater volume of bladder with retention of urine) | Bladder stimulation with contraction of bladder, relaxation of sphincter, (reduced bladder volume and tendency to elimination of urine; erection of penis) |

the synaptic space, stimulating acetylcholine receptors. The parasympathetic system is sometimes called the *cholinergic system;* it stimulates cholinergic receptors.

This leads to one of the most important concepts in psychopharmacology. Many psychotropic drugs (in fact, many drugs in general) are *anticholinergic.* This means that they interfere with the action of acetylcholine at its

receptor sites, usually by blocking access of the neurotransmitter to the receptor.

Understanding this concept immediately explains the
mechanism of some of the most common side effects of
many psychotropic drugs: blurred vision, dry mouth, constipation, difficulty with erection, or rapid heart.

For example, the *vagus nerve* is a large cranial nerve
which innervates the heart, stomach and other areas. It is a
parasympathetic, cholinergic nerve. It is in a state of mild,
continuous stimulation and exerts a slowing effect on the
heart, but speeds peristalsis, the motion of the intestinal
tract.

If a medication is administered which blocks the action
of acetylcholine, the effects of the vagus nerve will be
abolished or reduced. Moreover, the sympathetic innervation to the heart, intestinal tract and other organs will be
unopposed. This will result in a *speeding* of the heart rate
and a *slowing* of the intestinal tract. The patient may
complain of a rapid pulse and constipation. (It should be
added that sometimes, as in the case of a patient with
diarrhea, a slowing of the gut is the effect desired and an
anticholinergic agent will be given).

# CHAPTER 6

# NEUROTRANSMITTERS

$\mathbf{A}$T this point, the concept of neurotransmitters will be expanded. Neurotransmitters are those substances which transmit impulses between neurons in the brain and to tissue receptors in the peripheral nervous system. There are several neurotransmitters which have been well defined, but there are many others which are not so well defined; certainly many others which have not yet been discovered.

Neurotransmitters concentrate in specific areas of the brain. Tracts which mediate specific types of activity may utilize a specific neurotransmitter or several neurotransmitters. Thus, a tract in the brain may be called *dopaminergic,* if dopamine is the principal neurotransmitter.

Major known neurotransmitters include dopamine, norepinephrine, acetylcholine, and serotonin. Serotonin is one of a class of compounds called *indoleamines.* Dopamine, epinephrine and norepinephrine are classified as *catecholamines.* It is of some importance to become familiar with how these neurotransmitters are formed in the body. A review of this illustrates enzyme action and introduces the concept of *precursors.* Precursors are those substances which occur in the synthesis of neurotransmitters (and other compounds).

While the body's enzymes can synthesize much of what is needed by the organism, some compounds cannot be made by the system, and must be included in the diet or produced by the action of intestinal bacteria. *Phenylalanine,* an essential amino acid, is such a compound. It is taken in the diet and, among other possible metabolic pathways, becomes the neurotransmitter dopamine. It is important to emphasize that each step of the process of this catecholamine synthesis is enzyme-mediated:

Phenylalanine
↓         **Phenylalanine hydroxylase**
Tyrosine
↓         Tyrosine Hydroxylase
DOPA
↓         Aromatic-1-Amino Acid Decarboxylase
Dopamine*
↓         Dopamine-B-Hydroxylase
Norepinephrine*
↓         Phenylethanolamine-N-methyltransferase
Epinephrine*
↓

Normetanephrine

Vanillylmandelic Acid (VMA) - excreted in the urine

Phenylalanine, Tyrosine, and DOPA are *precursors* of dopamine.

Similarly, the amino acid tryptophan, taken in the diet, is the precursor of serotonin:

Tryptophan
↓         Tryptophan 5 hydroxylase
50H Tryptophan (5 hydroxytryptophan)
↓         Aromatic L-amino acid decarboxylase
Serotonin (5 hydroxytryptamine)
↓         Several steps of enzyme degradation, including
         MAO
50H Indoleacetic acid (the form in which it is excreted)

---

*These are the major *catecholamine neurotransmitters*. From this point on, they are metabolized to other products and eventually to the form in which excretion occurs.

The previously mentioned syntheses occur in the neurons themselves.

Acetylcholine, a neurotransmitter in the peripheral nervous system is also an important neurotransmitter in the brain.

It is not essential for the non-medical practitioner to memorize these syntheses. However, he should become familiar with the concept of neurotransmitter synthesis and the various categories of neurotransmitters.

# CHAPTER 7

# NEUROANATOMY

**P**ASSING from the molecular level to the anatomical, a discussion of basic neuroanatomy will be presented. Some knowledge of the structure and function of the brain and spinal cord is essential to the understanding of the actions of psychotropic drugs.

There is much more specific knowledge of how the drugs cause annoying side effects than how they exert desired antipsychotic, antidepressant and tranquilizing actions. But to understand the nature and seriousness of these side effects, it is necessary to have some understanding of normal neuroanatomy and neurophysiology.

The brain is composed of several anatomically separate areas: the *cortex,* the *midbrain,* the *cerebellum* and the *brain stem,* which extends into the spinal cord.

The following is a discussion of each area with special reference to those structures which are important in psychopharmacology. The discussion is by no means exhaustive; it hardly scratches the surface of the complex field of neuroanatomy. It is the fundamental information necessary to have some appreciation of drug action.

## The Cortex

The cortex is the mass of tissue covering the top, or *superior,* aspect of the brain. It is anatomically and, to some extent, functionally divided into masses or *lobes— frontal, temporal, parietal* and *occipital* (see Fig. 9). These lobes are further divided into mounds of tissue called *gyri* and separated by infoldings called *sulci.* Specific functions have been mapped in the lobes with the exception of the

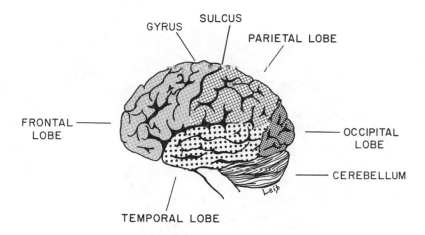

GYRUS SULCUS
PARIETAL LOBE
FRONTAL LOBE
OCCIPITAL LOBE
CEREBELLUM
TEMPORAL LOBE

LATERAL VIEW OF BRAIN
SHOWING MAJOR ANATOMICAL DIVISIONS

Figure 9.

frontal lobe. Frontal-lobe functions are not well defined, but it is generally agreed that personality traits, judgment, mood, foresight, and motor control are centered there.

The parietal, occipital, and temporal lobes are concerned with reception and conceptual elaboration of sensory data. The occipital lobe houses visual perception. The temporal lobes have to do with memory, auditory and taste phenomenon. Speech and language functions are centered in the parietal lobes and also, to some extent, in the temporal and frontal lobes.

At the highest or most superior area of the cortex, there are two strips of tissue separated by a deep sulcus. The strip toward the back of the head, or *posterior,* is called the sensory cortex. It is to this area that all incoming sensations from various body areas are relayed by structures deeper in the brain (see Fig. 10).

MOTOR CORTEX

SENSORY CORTEX

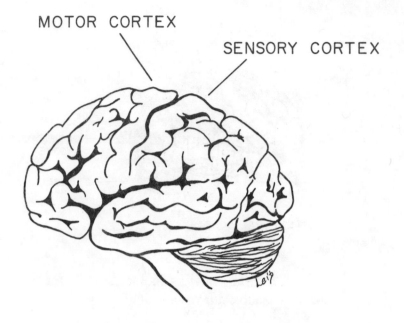

## LATERAL VIEW OF BRAIN
## SHOWING SENSORY & MOTOR CORTEX

Figure 10.

Just in front of, or *anterior,* to this area is the motor cortex. It is from this area that impulses stimulating voluntary motion originate. Each area of cortex is correlated with some specific portion of the body. The area of cortex controlling the body part is proportional in size to the amount of control and activity usual in that area. Thus, there is a large strip of motor cortex alloted to the hands, feet and face, areas characterized by precise motor control, and relatively little area for the abdomen.

Brain structures are paired. Both sides of the cortex are anatomically identical. They are connected by a structure, the *corpus callosum,* so impulses received in one hemisphere are transmitted to the opposite hemisphere. However, one hemisphere generally houses more highly developed functions than the other. This is *cerebral dominance.*

Usually, the dominant hemisphere determines handedness — generally a right-handed person has left cerebral dominance, and vice versa. An injury to the dominant side, by stroke or other trauma, is more disabling than one on the opposite side. However, in a very young person, functions may be fairly easily picked up by the opposite hemisphere, and recovery is more complete than in a mature individual.

Impulses from the motor cortex are carried to the spinal cord via tracts of tissue, the *pyramidal tracts* (see Fig. 11). These tracts carry impulses down through the brain, receiving input from various other structures described below. For some unknown evolutionary reason, the pyramidal tracts (and other tracts) cross over to the opposite side of the system. The tract which arises from the left motor cortex controls the right side of the body. After crossing, the pyramidal tracts descend in the spinal cord, its impulses reaching the roots of the spinal nerves via connecting neurons (see p. 26). Impulses carried by the spinal nerves eventually reach the muscles whose contractions cause the voluntary motion of limbs, trunk, and face (see Fig. 12).

## The Extrapyramidal System

A moment's reflection will show that there are other impulses which descend from the brain to the body muscles. The pyramidal tracts carry impulses from the consciously controlled motor cortex, but not all motion is

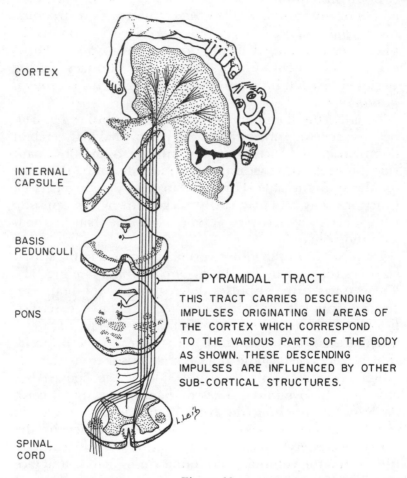

CORTEX

INTERNAL
CAPSULE

BASIS
PEDUNCULI

PONS

SPINAL
CORD

———— PYRAMIDAL TRACT

THIS TRACT CARRIES DESCENDING
IMPULSES ORIGINATING IN AREAS OF
THE CORTEX WHICH CORRESPOND
TO THE VARIOUS PARTS OF THE BODY
AS SHOWN. THESE DESCENDING
IMPULSES ARE INFLUENCED BY OTHER
SUB-CORTICAL STRUCTURES.

Figure 11.

voluntary. Little or no conscious effort is required to keep
an upright position, to walk, or to write.

A normal person performs many small accessory motions which are not conscious, but lend color and expression to volitional acts, such as facial expression, swinging
of the arms while walking, and small gestures. These *accessory movements*, which modify voluntary movements,

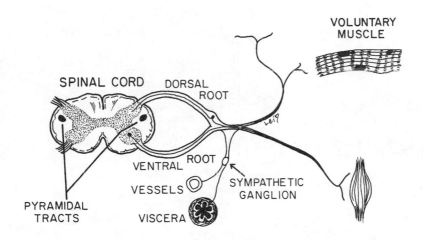

VOLUNTARY
MUSCLE

SPINAL CORD     DORSAL
                    ROOT

VENTRAL   ROOT

PYRAMIDAL
TRACTS

VESSELS

VISCERA

SYMPATHETIC
GANGLION

## SPINAL NERVES, ACTIVATED BY IMPULSES FROM THE PYRAMIDAL TRACTS, CONTROL VOLUNTARY MUSCLE.

Figure 12.

are influenced by a group of structures below the cortex. These structures are collectively known as the *extrapyramidal system.*

This refers to those structures which influence the pyramidal tract discharges exclusive of the cerebellum and balance apparatus (see below). Several of these structures, the *putamen, globus pallidus* and *caudate nucleus* are also known as the *basal ganglia,* or *corpus striatum* (see Fig. 13).

Other structures include the *substantia nigra* and the *reticular formation* of the brain stem (see Fig. 14.). The basal ganglia cluster around the *thalamus,* an egg-shaped mass of tissue which relays incoming data from the

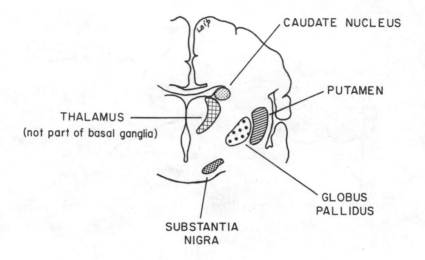

CAUDATE NUCLEUS

PUTAMEN

THALAMUS
(not part of basal ganglia)

GLOBUS
PALLIDUS

SUBSTANTIA
NIGRA

CROSS-SECTION OF BRAIN
SHOWING BASAL GANGLIA

Figure 13.

peripheral system to various parts of the brain. Almost all incoming data from the environment is relayed through the thalamus.

Although the above material may seem confusing and esoteric, it is relevant to the understanding of some of the major side effects of antipsychotic medication. For example, one of the major neurotransmitters in the extrapyramidal system is dopamine; another is acetylcholine. When there is damage to the dopaminergic tracts in this system, a condition exists known as Parkinson's disease.

This disease is characterized by a masklike face with little change in facial expression and decreased eye blinking. There is rigidity of the arms with a distinctive

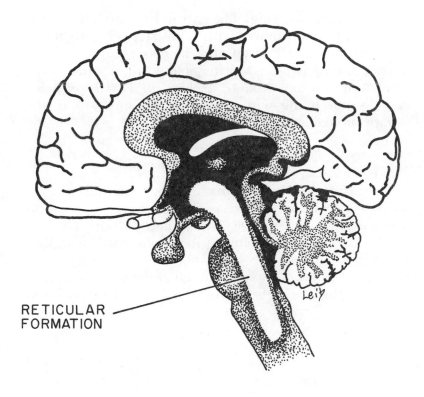

RETICULAR
FORMATION

# RETICULAR  FORMATION

## FILTER FOR INCOMING & OUTGOING DATA

Figure 14.

*cogwheel rigidity*: When the arm is passively bent, the examiner will feel an alternate tightening and letting go of the forearm. When the hands are at rest, there may be a tremor with motion similar to those employed in rolling a pill. This tremor disappears when the hand is voluntarily moved. There also may be a characteristic shuffling gait

with little arm-swinging. The patient has difficulty beginning to move and moves with small steps, but then has
difficulty stopping himself after he gets going.

This disease is described in some detail, because some
psychotropic drugs produce a *chemical Parkinson's disease,* by interfering with dopamine transmission in the
extrapyramidal system.

### Cerebellum

The basic sensations of touch, pain, heat, and cold are
familiar to everyone. There is another form of sensation
which is in continuous use. This is the sensation of aware-
ness of the position of the various body parts, a feeling
which is not exactly any of the above. This sensory input
is *proprioception.* Although it is felt at the cortical area, so
that it is possible to be aware of a body part's position,

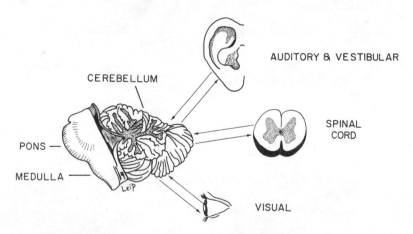

CEREBELLUM CORRELATES SENSORY INPUT
TO COORDINATE MOVEMENT

Figure 15.

proprioceptive input is most important in the cerebellum.

The cerebellum is located below the cortex at the back of the brain (see Fig. 15). It receives input from the spinal cord, as well as from visual, auditory, balance control (vestibular), and cortical portions of the brain. The cerebellum coordinates movement correlating visual and positional data so that motions are smooth and direct. A minute analysis of any movement, e.g. moving a forkful of food from plate to mouth, will show that it is actually made up of many tiny movements continually corrected relative to desired direction and speed, much as the guidance system of a missile constantly corrects its course.

Damage to the cerebellum results in a loss of this smooth control. A patient with such damage, while not paralyzed, must consciously direct his every muscular action, continually correcting for error. This results in clumsy, faltering, jerky movement.

The most common drug-induced damage to the cerebellum is by alcohol. Its effects on the cerebellum cause the typical drunken gait, slurred speech, impaired balance, and poor dexterity of the intoxicated person. Barbiturates, another psychotropic drug group, have this effect, as do other drugs to be discussed.

## The Midbrain and Limbic System

On the inner-lower surface of the cerebral hemispheres, there is a group of structures which have come in for a great deal of attention as the action of some tranquilizing drugs has been clarified. The limbic area, in primitive animals, has to do mainly with the *olfactory,* or smelling, function. In man, however, its functions apparently include emotion, recent memory, approach and avoidance behavior, and some control of sympathetic and parasympathetic activity. The limbic system is also closely connected to the *hypothalamus,* a group of nuclei which exert some control over the pituitary gland, the master gland of the endocrine system (see p. 51).

In 1937, Papez, in a paper entitled "A Proposed Mechanism of Emotion," hypothesized that neural circuitry, involving the limbic system, the thalamus, the hypothalamus, and the cortex formed a reverberating circuit responsible for the persistence of emotion and its coloring of other brain processes. Further studies have supported this hypothesis.

The structures of the limbic system include the *amygdala, septum, mammillary bodies, fornix, hippocampus,*

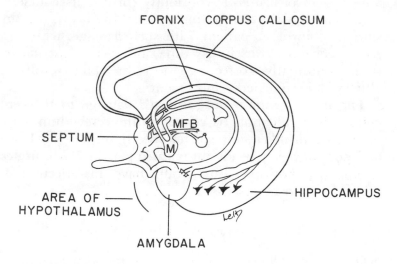

**LIMBIC SYSTEM**

Figure 16.

*medial forebrain bundle,* and other minor structures. These terms frequently appear in literature dealing with tranquilizing medications (see Fig. 16).

## The Reticular Formation

The reticular formation is a difficult area to define anatomically. It extends from the thalamus down through the medulla, which is in the lower brain stem. As mentioned above, the thalamus is the relay point for incoming sensory data. The reticular formation may be considered as a filter for incoming data. It also influences impulses flowing out of the brain to the spinal cord, descending data (see Fig. 17).

The reticular formation mediates arousal, wakefulness, and attention. It influences muscle control. It integrates

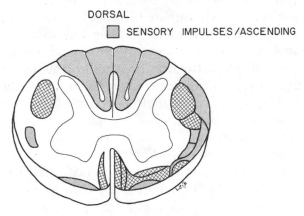

DORSAL

□ SENSORY IMPULSES/ASCENDING

▨ MOTOR IMPULSES/DESCENDING

VENTRAL

**SPINAL CORD SHOWING**
**ASCENDING-DESCENDING CONDUCTION PATHWAYS**

Figure 17.

sensory input, functioning to screen out input which may
be irrelevant to the organism's functioning.

Both acetylcholine and epinephrine are found in different areas and in different amounts in the reticular formation. It may be the site of action of LSD and
amphetamines, as these drugs produce distortions of
normal attention. Schizophrenia is considered by some to
be a disorder in which the patient has difficulty separating
relevant from irrelevant data in his environment. It has
been hypothesized that an abnormality in the reticular
formation plays a role in this disease.

### Spinal Cord

All of the above portions of the brain, and many not
discussed, influence the impulses which eventually im-
pinge on the spinal cord. Some of these neural impulses
are consciously initiated from the cortex. Others are under
control of lower levels, and regulate such automatic activities as breathing, blood pressure, and antigravity postural
control. All influences eventually flow to a final common
pathway, ending on a group of muscle fibers.

The spinal cord itself is a complex structure, housing
ascending and descending conduction pathways, and
reflex neurons. Generally, the posterior section of the
spinal cord, or *dorsal* area, carries ascending *sensory* impulses. The anterior, or *ventral* portion, carries descending
impulses which mediate muscle movement (see Fig. 17).

* * *

In the subsequent sections on drugs, some neurological
side effects will be discussed. The information in this section is the necessary background to these discussions, and
the discussions will amplify the information in this section.

However, this material on neuroanatomy and neurophysiology should not conclude without an additional word of caution. The information given is only a basic outline of the fundamentals necessary to begin to understand psychopharmacology. It would be an error for the reader to consider himself informed on the subject even after absorbing all of the presentation. The same holds true for all the sections on anatomy and physiology, but especially for this one.

CHAPTER 8

# NEUROPHYSIOLOGY
# AND ENDOCRINOLOGY

THIS section will cover those aspects of
endocrinology and neurophysiology which relate to the
actions and side effects of psychotropic drugs.

The endocrine system is a group of glands which secrete
substances regulating body metabolism. These metabolic
regulators are designated *hormones*. The organs which
secrete them include the thyroid, parathyroid, pancreas,
adrenal glands, testicles, ovaries, and others. Hormone
secretion is partially regulated by the *pituitary gland,*
which secretes substances which stimulate or inhibit the
various endocrine glands.

The pituitary gland, in turn, is influenced by the *hypothalamus.* It is at the hypothalamic-pituitary axis that
many psychotropic drugs exert their endocrine effects.
There are dopaminergic and other neurotransmitter connections between the pituitary and the hypothalamus (see
Fig. 18).

## The Hypothalamus

The hypothalamus is a portion of the midbrain below
the thalamus. It is composed of structural subgroups
called nuclei, which have specific connections with various other parts of the brain, especially the limbic system.
It also has both neural and vascular connections with the
pituitary gland (see Fig. 19).

The hypothalamic nuclei influence regulatory mechanisms of the body. Hypothalamic stimulation affects a wide

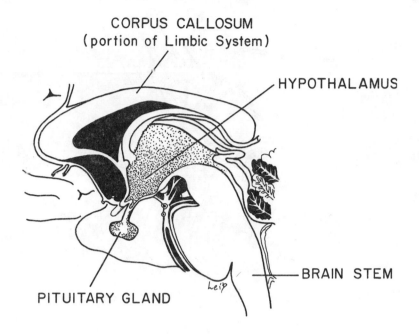

CORPUS CALLOSUM
(portion of Limbic System)

HYPOTHALAMUS

BRAIN STEM

PITUITARY GLAND

## MIDBRAIN & BRAINSTEM
### LIMBIC-HYPOTHALAMIC-PITUITARY RELATIONSHIPS

Figure 18.

variety of functions, including temperature regulation, appetite, sexual behavior, defensive reactions, growth, milk secretion, pleasure, satiety, hunger, and sleep. The hypothalamus also exerts some influence on the autonomic nervous system. Stimulation of various areas may cause both sympathetic and parasympathetic response.

### The Pituitary Gland

In order to appreciate the actions of the hypothalamus,

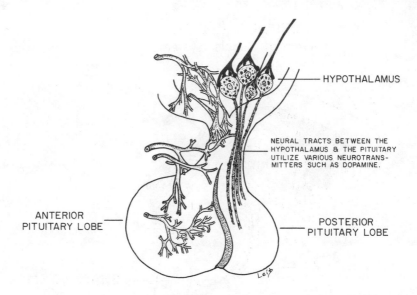

HYPOTHALAMUS

NEURAL TRACTS BETWEEN THE
HYPOTHALAMUS & THE PITUITARY
UTILIZE VARIOUS NEUROTRANS-
MITTERS SUCH AS DOPAMINE.

ANTERIOR
PITUITARY LOBE

POSTERIOR
PITUITARY LOBE

VASCULAR & NEURAL HYPOTHALAMIC-PITUITARY CONNECTIONS

Figure 19.

it is necessary to understand the anatomy and physiology of the pituitary gland. It is located at the end of a stalk below the hypothalamus and is divided into three lobes; the *anterior, posterior* and a small *intermediate lobe* (see Fig. 20).

The anterior lobe secretes hormones which stimulate the thyroid gland (TSH - thyrotropin), adrenal glands (ACTH - corticotropin), growth hormone (GH - somatotropin), ovaries (FSH - follicle stimulating hormone), and milk ducts of the breast and the placenta (prolactin and luteo-tropin).

The posterior lobe secretes a hormone which regulates the concentration of salts in the body fluids. It is called *antidiuretic hormone* (ADH), because it influences the kidney to reduce urine production, and to concentrate the

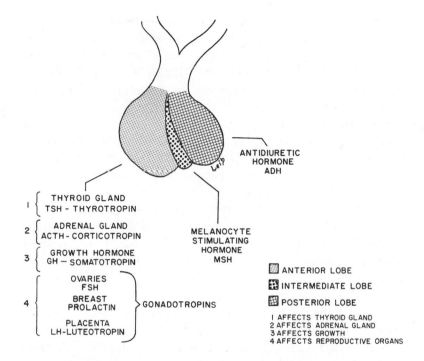

THYROID GLAND
TSH - THYROTROPIN

ADRENAL GLAND
ACTH - CORTICOTROPIN

GROWTH HORMONE
GH – SOMATOTROPIN

OVARIES
FSH

BREAST
PROLACTIN

PLACENTA
LH-LUTEOTROPIN

GONADOTROPINS

ANTIDIURETIC
HORMONE
ADH

MELANOCYTE
STIMULATING
HORMONE
MSH

ANTERIOR LOBE
INTERMEDIATE LOBE
POSTERIOR LOBE

I AFFECTS THYROID GLAND
2 AFFECTS ADRENAL GLAND
3 AFFECTS GROWTH
4 AFFECTS REPRODUCTIVE ORGANS

PITUITARY GLAND  LOBES, HORMONES & TARGET HORMONES

Figure 20.

urine. A lack of this hormone results in excretion of large volumes of dilute urine. A patient with this condition would need to consume much more water than normal. This disease, diabetes insipidus, can result from injury to the posterior pituitary, part of the hypothalamus, or disruption of the neural connections between the posterior pituitary and the hypothalamus. The posterior pituitary also secretes *oxytocin,* a hormone which causes milk ejection.

The intermediate lobe secretes a hormone which stimulates cells, *melanocytes,* which in turn secrete the skin pigment *melanin.* This hormone is called *melanocyte stimulating hormone* (MSH).

The hypothalamus influences both anterior and posterior pituitary secretion. Anterior pituitary secretion is controlled by hypothalamic hormones which reach the anterior lobe via a special circulatory system. Posterior pituitary regulation is achieved by direct neural connections (see Fig. 19).

The hypothalamic substances which regulate pituitary hormone output are *releasing and inhibiting* hormones. The importance of this hypothalamic-pituitary relationship is that sensory impressions, which reach the brain from the environment, and emotional states, influence the hypothalamus, which in turn affects the pituitary. The system's endocrine glands then respond, causing changes in the body's physiological state. This may explain such phenomenon as loss of appetite during depression, disruption of the menstrual cycle during stress, or increased urination during anxiety attacks.

More to the point of this text is that various psychotropic drugs influence the working of the neuroendocrine system. These side effects will be discussed, where appropriate, using the above information as background.

# CHAPTER 9

# THE HEART

**A** BRIEF presentation of a few points of cardiac physiology will clear the way to understand some effects of psychotropic drugs on the heart.

The heart is a four-chamber pump made of muscle. Blood enters the thin-walled *atria,* the top chambers, and passes through valves into the thick-walled *ventricles,* the bottom chambers (see Fig. 21).

The pumping action is stimulated by an excitatory wave which smoothly passes over the cardiac muscle, causing the fibers to contract rhythmically, and in coordination

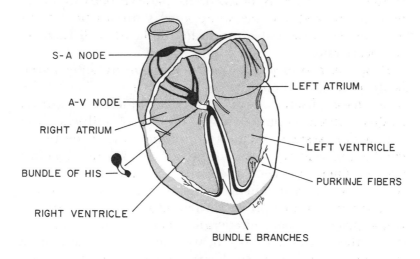

SCHEMATIC OF HEART
SHOWING CONDUCTION SYSTEM

Figure 21.

with each other. (Obviously, if muscle fibers were to contract irregularly, in an uncoordinated manner, efficient pumping would be impossible.) A state of cardiac contraction is designated *systole*. Relaxation (and the heart is in a state of complete relaxation most of the time) is called *diastole*. The heart tissue itself is nourished by a system of vessels called coronary arteries. Blockage of a coronary artery may cause injury or death to the cardiac tissue it supplies, a condition termed *myocardial infarction*.

The wave of excitation which causes contraction of the heart is propagated over a specialized conduction system (see Fig. 21). The excitatory wave originates at the *sinoatrial node*, passes to the *atrial-ventricular node* and so over the ventricles through the *Bundle of His*. This conduction system is influenced by the vagus nerve. Stimulation of the vagus will result in a slowing of the heart rate. If the vagus nerve is blocked, its parasympathetic effect will be reduced and the unopposed sympathetic, adrenergic nerves, which also innervate the heart, will increase the heart rate.

Drugs may influence the nerves to the heart; an example is atropine, an anticholinergic drug. Drugs may affect the heart tissue itself; one is digitalis, which strengthens cardiac muscle contractions. A drug may influence the conduction system, such as quinidine, which decreases conduction velocity. Some drugs are adrenergic blocking agents. There are beta-adrenergic receptors in the heart which, when stimulated, increase heart rate and the strength of contraction of cardiac muscle. Some psychotropic drugs are beta-adrenergic blockers, and so may reduce the efficiency of heart function. They may simultaneously speed the heart, however, by their anticholinergic effect on the vagus nerve.

The effects of psychotropic drugs on the heart may show up on the electrocardiogram. This is a tracing of the electrical activity of the heart. Different parts of the tracing indicate activity in different parts of the heart. The literature is replete with such phrases as *the lengthening of the ST segment, prolongation of the QT and PR intervals,* and *blunting of T-waves.* In general, these may be understood as referring to the interference by the psychotropic drug on electrical conduction in the heart. There may also be a direct depressant effect on cardiac muscle.

# CHAPTER 10

# THE EYE

Some of the most troublesome, and potentially dangerous, side effects of psychotropic drugs have to do with the eye. A brief review of ocular anatomy and physiology is necessary to understand these side effects.

As discussed above, the pupil of the eye dilates when sympathetically stimulated, and contracts when parasympathetically stimulated. It also dilates if parasympathetic blockade occurs due to an anticholinergic drug. In order to understand the mechanism of dilatation and constriction, the basic anatomy of the eye must be reviewed (see Fig. 22).

The *iris*, the pigmented portion of the eye, controls the amount of light entering through the lens. When looking at objects over twenty feet away, the light rays passing through the lens are essentially parallel, and the lens focuses them on the retina. The *retina* may be considered as a group of specialized nerve endings which convey visual impulses to the brain where image recognition occurs. When focusing on an object closer than twenty feet, the lens must change its shape in order to keep the retinal image sharp.

A circular muscular body, the *ciliary muscle*, contracts, thereby allowing the lens to assume a more convex shape. This bends the light rays more and brings the new image into retinal focus (see Fig. 23). Simultaneously, the iris contracts a little. This process, the thickening of the lens and the contraction of the pupil, is called *accommodation*. It is caused by the action of cholinergic nerves to the eye. Some psychotropic drugs produce partial or complete paralysis of accommodation. The patient complains of blurred vision, especially when reading or doing other close work.

The anterior portion of the eye is divided by the iris into two chambers. The anterior chamber is filled with a clear fluid, the *aqueous humor*, which is derived from the plasma and in a continuous state of formation, circulation, and

58

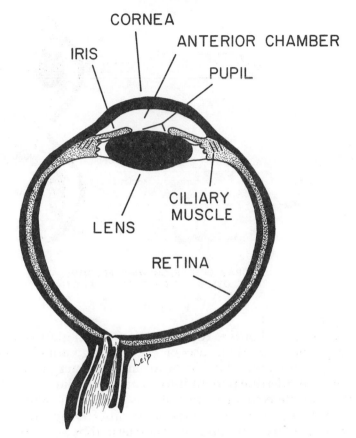

CORNEA

ANTERIOR CHAMBER

IRIS

PUPIL

CILIARY
MUSCLE

LENS

RETINA

## LONGITUDINAL SECTION
## THROUGH THE MIDDLE OF THE EYE

Figure 22.

excretion. Sometimes an excess amount of this fluid is formed, or there is a disorder of the mechanism for its drainage from the anterior chamber. This condition is called *glaucoma*. In this condition the buildup of fluid in the eye may result in pressure damage to the retina.

When the pupil is contracted, drainage of the aqueous humor is improved. Conversely, when it is dilated, drainage

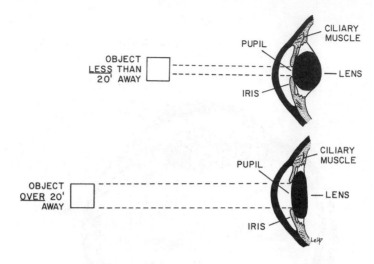

DIAGRAM OF EYE SHOWING ACCOMMODATION
TO CLOSE & FAR OBJECTS RESPECTIVELY

Figure 23.

is hampered. For this reason, patients with glaucoma must be cautious in their use of eye-dilating, anticholinergic drugs. Moreover, the use of an anticholinergic drug may push a borderline patient into an attack of glaucoma. There is a two percent incidence of this disease in patients over forty. Glaucoma is often gradual in onset. Drug-precipitated attacks are usually sudden, characterized by agonizing pain and blurring of vision, and often accompanied by nausea and vomiting.

Psychotropic medications may also affect the retina. Retinal changes can only be detected by instrument examination, but the patient's complaints may alert the practitioner that an examination is necessary. Some complaints to be watched for are blurring of vision, a decrease in night vision, and "specks" before the eyes. Ideally, patients on anticholinergic and certain other psychotropic drugs should have regular complete physical exams. This is, unfortunately, uncommon in actual practice.

# CHAPTER 11

# ALLERGY

## "Allergy" vs "Side Effect"

PATIENTS will often say that they are "allergic" to a certain drug, or group of drugs. This statement should not be accepted without further questioning. *Allergy* is a specific term, indicating that the system has developed antibodies against an antigen, in this case a drug. However, a patient will often call a side effect an allergy.

A patient may claim allergy to codeine because of stomach upset, a common side effect. Some patients mistake the dry mouth and neurological side effects of the major tranquilizers for allergies. If the practitioner accepts the patient's report without question, he risks withholding an important drug from the patient.

On the other hand, a genuine allergy is a potential danger. This dilemma can usually be resolved by carefully questioning the patient. He should be asked to describe his "allergy." A genuine allergy may be represented by a rash, hives, generalized itching, wheezing, difficulty in breathing, diarrhea, swelling of the face, hands and feet, fainting, or other serious physical signs.

The mode of administration of the drug may determine the strength of allergic response. Orally ingested drugs seldom produce clinically serious allergic response, whereas injected drugs do. (It is also necessary to distinguish allergic shock from needle phobia.)

## How Allergies Occur

This section will describe the way in which allergies

develop, and the mechanisms underlying allergic reactions. As will be seen, understanding a few basic principles explains a wide variety of allergic reactions.

Drug allergy is a special class of allergy. An *allergy* is defined as an altered response to a specific stimulus. The body reacts to a foreign substance in a way which disrupts normal physiological function.

Drug allergy occurs when a drug becomes an *antigen*. An antigen is defined as a substance which stimulates the formation of *antibodies*. An example of this is the formation of antibodies to a bacteria or virus. The body produces a substance, the antibody, which combines with the antigen, a virus or microbe, either rendering it physiologically inert or permitting other body defenses to destroy it. An example of the latter is engulfment and destruction of bacteria by the white blood cells. This process, *phagocytosis,* may be facilitated by the presence of an antibody on the surface of the bacteria. The antigen-antibody response is basic to the immunological system vital to protection against disease-causing organisms.

No one is allergic to a drug the first time it is administered, although if there is an allergy to a chemically similar drug, a *cross sensitization* may occur. The body must have time to respond to the drug-antigen with the formation of antibodies. When the drug is administered again, a mild allergic reaction may occur. On repeated administration, the allergic reaction may become progressively more severe as antibody formation continues, and the antibodies spread through the system and permeate organ tissue.

As discussed above, when a drug enters the circulation, it becomes attached to plasma proteins (see p. 13). Its metabolites, as they form by enzymatic action, also attach to plasma proteins. It is in this protein-bound form that the drug becomes antigenic. (It should be reemphasized that usually it does not become antigenic.) The drug, or drug metabolite, attaches to a plasma protein. A small and well-defined portion of the molecule then becomes the antigenic determinant. Antigens and antibodies are specific, much as a key is to a lock. They will react only with each other or compounds almost exactly alike in structure.

The next step of the allergic process occurs when the drug-plasma protein antigen is exposed to lymphoid tissue. Almost all compounds eventually pass through the lymphatic circulation where they encounter *lymph nodes.* These are masses of tissue in which populations of white blood cells called *lymphocytes* reside. There are various subtypes of lymphocytes, but the important point is that they differentiate into cells which produce antibodies. These antibodies then enter the general circulation, as part of the plasma protein.

Another form of antibody activity is the production of a type of cell which acts itself like an antibody. This type of response, while it can occur with drugs, is uncommon with psychotropic drugs and will not be discussed further.

## The Basic Allergic Response

The stage is now set for an allergic response. All allergic responses are basically due to the combination of an antigen and an antibody. The severity and type of response is determined by where it takes place and how much or what tissue is involved.

If the patient now receives another dose of the antigenic drug, it attaches to plasma protein and eventually combines with the waiting antibody. If the antibody is attached to the surface of a cell, the chemical combination of antigen with antibody damages the cell membrane. The disruption of cell membrane results in the release of a compound, *histamine,* from certain cell types.

Histamine causes several important reactions which result in the clinically observable allergic response. It causes dilatation of blood vessels, contraction of smooth muscle, such as found in bronchi and intestine, and increased permeability of capillary walls, permitting the escape of fluid into surrounding tissues. It also causes the sensation of itching.

There are other substances besides histamine released by antigen-antibody reactions, such as serotonin, bradykinan, and acetylcholine. They cause such responses as pain, constriction of large blood vessels, and smooth muscle contraction.

With the above in mind, it is possible to understand some allergic phenomenon. At a local level, the release of histamine causes the swelling, redness, and itching characteristic of *hives*. A massive systemic antibody response results in a condition called *anaphylactic shock*. Massive capillary permeability and vasodilatation causes a drop in effective blood volume and lowered blood pressure. Passage of fluid into tissue results in swelling, or *edema* in the face, hands or feet. Constriction of smooth muscle of the bronchi and larynx results in wheezing and choking. In the intestine, vomiting and diarrhea is the result of gut muscle contraction. Anaphylaxis is potentially fatal, but most allergic reactions are milder.

Another form of allergy is called *serum sickness*. In contrast to anaphylaxis, this reaction usually occurs two to seven days following drug ingestion. It is characterized by fever, edema, and large patches of hives, or *urticaria*. There also may be a rash and enlargement of the lymph nodes.

### Blood Dyscrasias

The allergic or toxic effects of drugs on the hematologic (blood) system result in conditions called *blood dyscrasias*. Since many types of psychotropic drugs may provoke these important responses, the blood dyscrasias will be described in some detail.

### Agranulocytosis

Agranulocytosis is the condition in which there is reduced or no bone marrow production of a type of white cell called *polymorphonuclear leukocytes*. These cells function to destroy bacteria. Their absence leads to highly increased susceptibility to infection. The patient may develop severe ulcerative lesions on mucosal surfaces, such as the mouth and throat. This can lead to an overwhelming bacterial infection and death. For this reason, a patient taking a drug who develops fever and sore throat should have an immediate blood count.

In fact, blood counts every six months should be done routinely on all patients who are regularly taking most psychotropic drugs. In this way, early drops in white blood cell count can be detected before clinical signs appear. Stopping the medication will usually halt the blood dyscrasia. The patient may then be changed to another drug which has similar therapeutic effect, but to which he is not allergic.

### Leukopenia

Leukopenia refers to suppression of all white blood cell types. Its symptoms are similar to agranulocytosis.

### Eosinophilia

Eosinophilia means an increased number of a type of white cell, *eosinophil*. These cells tend to migrate into tissues in which antigen-antibody reactions take place. An increased eosinophil count is an indication that an allergic condition exists.

### Purpura

A purpura is literally an area of skin discoloration. This

can occur in a number of conditions other than allergy, such as severe bacterial infection leading to destruction of blood vessels and bleeding into the skin. A bruise caused by trauma may also be considered a kind of purpura. A drug allergy, however, may cause the destruction of a type of blood cell, *platelets* or *thrombocytes*. These tiny cells are important in the process of blood coagulation. When the platelet count drops, due to drug allergy, bleeding into the skin and other organs may occur. This is a potentially serious condition, but remits if the offending agent is withdrawn. When purpura is caused by platelet decrease, it is termed *thrombocytopenic purpura*.

## Pancytopenia

Pancytopenia is the term reserved for the depression of all blood cell types. All of the above clinical features may be present, and the patient may die of hemorrhage and infection.

## Anemia

Anemia means a reduction in hemoglobin, due to allergic bone marrow depression, or the destruction of red cells by antigen-antibody reactions on the cell wall. This condition is known as *hemolytic anemia,* because the red cells *lyse,* or dissolve. The symptoms and signs of anemia include fatigue, breathlessness, and pallor. Since fatigue, breathlessness, and pallor can also be psychogenic, only laboratory testing can truly diagnose the condition.

Allergic reactions may also damage other organ systems, such as the liver and kidneys. In the skin, allergy-related phenomena may result in extreme sensitivity to sunlight, with resulting sunburn. These conditions will be discussed in greater detail along with the drugs with which they are most commonly associated.

# Part II
# Psychiatric Drugs

# CHAPTER 12

# A GENERAL SURVEY OF
# PSYCHOTROPIC DRUGS

THIS chapter is intended as a general overview of the types and uses of psychotropic drugs. It will also cover the diagnostic entities for which the various drugs are used.

There are two sources of information about drugs with which every mental health worker should be familiar. They are the Physician's Desk Reference (PDR), and drug package inserts.

The PDR is a yearly publication sent to all physicians. It is a catalogue of most of the available drugs in the United States, with more than 2500 entries and a product identification section in which several hundred drugs are pictured.

Each drug write-up gives the description of the drug, the indications for its use, the contraindications (when it should not be used), warnings, precautions, adverse effects, dosages, in what form the drug is supplied (pill, liquid, or injectable ampules), treatment of overdosage, and other pertinent information.

The drug write-up in the PDR is generally the same as that given in the insert included in every package of the drug. The insert may contain updated information not yet in the PDR.

The non-medical mental health worker who reads the package insert or PDR may be confused by the mass of information given. However, using this text as a background, he should be able to understand why the drug is used, the mechanisms of some side effects, and how it may be administered. The many side effects and dangers listed in the package insert may cause the worker to wonder why such a potentially dangerous substance is ever given at all.

The reality is that while some side effects, e.g. dry mouth, are very common, most are rare. Medico-legal considerations dictate that every side effect encountered should be listed in the drug write-up even if it has occurred only a few times in the thousands of patients to whom the drug has been given.

With experience, the mental health worker will learn which side effects are commonly complained of, and acquire some perspective about psychotropic drugs. This perspective should combine a sense of their immense value with an informed vigilance about potential adverse effects. He should be able to reassure, explain to the patient the side effects he may have, and be alert to possibly dangerous reactions. Such reactions must be passed on to the prescribing physician.

## SURVEY OF DRUGS

### Major Tranquilizers

The term "major tranquilizers" refers to that class of psychotropic drugs used to treat *psychotic disorders* — schizophrenia, manic-depressive psychosis, and psychotic depression. This class of drugs is also known as the *neuroleptics*. Psychosis is characterized by thought disorder, and does not necessarily imply a state of emotional agitation. Therefore, the term *tranquilizer* is somewhat misleading. Some major tranquilizers will bring the patient out of a state of immobility and withdrawal; many of the major tranquilizers have little actual tranquilizing effect.

There are several groups of antipsychotic drugs differentiated by their basic chemical structure. It is of little value for the practitioner to know the chemical structure. It is clinically true that the patient who does not respond well to one type of major tranquilizer may do well on one of a chemically different class. At present, there is no way to predict which patient will do well with what drug. There are some rough guidelines in terms of the degree of sedation produced, the incidence and kind of side effects, and possible concomitant antidepressant effect.

## Phenothiazines

This is the oldest class of major tranquilizers. The first, chlorpromazine (Thorazine®), was discovered in 1952 by Delay and Deniker, who were searching for a new antihistamine.

The phenothiazines revolutionized the treatment of schizophrenia. They were the first drugs which affected the thought disorder characteristic of that disease. They relieve paranoid feelings, hallucinations, delusions, and inability to distinguish relevant from irrelevant environmental data. They are useful in the manic phase of manic-depressive psychosis, and may be used in nonpsychotic states of anxiety and agitation. However, because of their potentially serious side effects, they are generally not regularly used in neurotic, as opposed to psychotic, conditions.

Examples of the phenothiazines are Thorazine (chlorpromazine), Mellaril® (thioridazine), Stelazine® (trifluoperizine), and Trilafon® (perphenizine).

## Butyrophenones

The butyrophenones are another class of major tranquilizers, with uses similar to the phenothiazines. The major example is Haldol® (haloperidol). This drug seems to be especially useful in geriatric patients.

## Thioxanthines

The thioxanthines are mainly represented by Navane®

(thiothixene). This drug may have an antidepressant as well as an antipsychotic effect.

Moban® (molindone) and Loxitane® (loxapine) are two major tranquilizers which are chemically different from those already in use. However, the actions and side effects of all the major tranquilizers are similar and will be discussed in detail in the chapter on phenothiazines.

There are several drugs which are given with major tranquilizers to reduce neurological side effects. Examples of these are the antiparkinsonian drugs Cogentin® (benztropine) and Artane® (trihexphenidyl). They are given to relieve the parkinsonian side effects of the major tranquilizers. They are themselves anticholinergic and so do not relieve dry mouth and constipation. The patient, therefore, is usually advised to drink frequently, chew gum, and to take bran or an occasional laxative for constipation.

## Minor Tranquilizers

These drugs are used to control anxiety and produce some sedation. Many are excellent sleep medications. They are generally used as adjuncts in the treatment of the neuroses, states in which anxiety is usually a central symptom.

The *barbiturates* were once used extensively as antianxiety drugs, but are not used much now because of their addictive potential, their suppression of cortical activity, and the possible fatal result of overdose. They retain the advantage of being cheap, however. Phenobarbital, a long-acting barbiturate, is not especially addicting. The shorter-acting barbiturates, such as Seconal® (amobarbital) are particularly addicting.

The *benzodiazepine* group is the most popular in clinical use today. It includes Valium® (diazepam), Librium® (chlordiazepoxide), Serax® (oxazepam), and Tranxene® (clorazepate). These drugs have a calming effect and, in some patients, produce mild euphoria. However, some patients may find themselves more depressed when taking them. For years they were considered non-addicting, but severe withdrawal reactions, including seizures, have been observed in patients who took large doses of Valium over a long period. Ideally, the minor tranquilizers should be taken only on an as-needed (p.r.n.) basis. Unlike the psychotic and depressive disorders, anxiety states are usually acute and intermittent, rather than chronic. Therefore, the minor tranquilizers should be taken only when needed, rather than regularly day after day.

Miltown® (Equanil®; meprobamate) is an older minor tranquilizer, prescribed much less since the advent of Valium and Librium. It is potentially addictive and may enhance depression. However, some patients prefer it over the more benign benzodiazepines, and it is also a good sleep medication.

*Atarax®* and the almost identical *Vistaril®* (hydroxyzine) are minor tranquilizers which have some autonomic side effects. For this reason, they are less pleasant to take and, therefore, are less potentially addicting. They have been found particularly useful in psychosomatic disorders. They are also of value for patients who are addiction-prone.

Benadryl® (diphenhydramine) and Phenergan® (promethazine) are used mainly as antihistamines (see p. 63). However, they are good sedative drugs and are occasionally so used. Benadryl may also be employed as an anti-parkinsonian agent for relief of side effects with the major tranquilizers.

## Antidepressants

Antidepressant medications are not stimulants. While they may relieve a patient of the torture and despair of depression, they do not generally induce euphoria. It may be said that they "bring the patient from the basement to the ground floor, but no higher."

There are two main groups of antidepressants, the *tricyclics*, and the *monoamine oxidase inhibitors* (MAOI's). The tricyclic antidepressants are by far the more widely used because of their relative safety.

Depressions may be divided into those which have a clear cause, e.g. the death of a loved one, and those which seem to have no clear precipitant and are prolonged. The former group is termed *exogenous* depression, the latter group *endogenous*. Some individuals seem to be depression-prone, possibly because of a genetic predisposition. It is possible that the tricyclics may correct an imbalance in brain neurotransmitters, which results in endogenous depression. A tendency to this imbalance may be hereditary and brought out by environmental factors.

Antidepressant drugs must be taken for extended periods, days to weeks, before they exert their full effect. The dosage must also be carefully regulated. A patient may not respond to, for example, 200 mg per day, but feel much better with 250 mg.

In addition to their antidepressant effect, some tricyclics also have a tranquilizing effect. The most sedative is Sinequan® (doxepin). Elavil® (amitriptyline) is also tranquilizing, but Tofranil® (imipramine) is not. Norpramin® (desipramine) may have a slight stimulant effect; Vivactil® (protriptyline) is quite stimulant and may induce anxiety in susceptible patients.

The monamine oxidase inhibitors, such as Marplan® (isocarboxazide), Nardil® (phenelzine), and Parnate® (tranylcypromine) are little-used because of their potentially serious side effects. Their mechanism of action will be discussed in the chapter on antidepressants.

## Stimulant Drugs

Stimulant drugs are not much used in psychiatric practice. The main stimulant drugs are the amphetamines and

Ritalin® (methylphenidate). Ritalin may be used as a mild stimulant in geriatric cases, to increase activity and cause a feeling of well-being. It may also be used in cases of drug-induced immobility, which is sometimes encountered with major tranquilizer therapy.

The main psychiatric use of the stimulant drug Ritalin is in the treatment of *minimal brain dysfunction* (MBD), the hyperactive syndrome of childhood. It causes a reduction in hyperactivity; the net behavioral effect is sedation, not stimulation.

The amphetamines are used in general medicine to reduce appetite. They also cause euphoria and increased energy. When the patient discontinues use, depression may ensue. This may lead to resuming the amphetamines, and habituation is formed. (*Habituation* should be distinguished. from *addiction*. Addiction means that the body physiology has adapted to the drug, and discontinuation may lead to measurable physiological withdrawal effects, such as alterations in consciousness, neuromuscular irritability, vomiting, rapid heart rate, and seizures. Habituation refers to a reward to the user in terms of euphoria, energy, or less depression, which then leads to continuation of use. There are not physical consequences to discontinuing the drug. *Tolerance* to a drug means that greater and greater amounts must be taken to produce the same effect. Thus, the amphetamines are habituating. Heroin is both habituating and addicting, and tolerance occurs.)

## Lithium

This is the first psychotropic drug which can be used to prevent a psychiatric illness before it happens. Lithium is employed in manic-depressive psychosis. In many patients with this disease, though not all, it stops the manic phase, by relieving such symptoms as extreme hyperactivity, sleeplessness, grandiosity, defective judgment, and unrealistic euphoria. When taken prophylactically in proper dosage, it prevents recurrence of manic attacks. It may also, though less predictably, prevent the depressed phase of this disease. It is necessary to monitor blood levels of lithium, as the therapeutic range is very close to the toxic level.

## Other Drugs

There are new psychoactive drugs coming on the market every year. Most of them fit into one of the above classes, and do not represent a significant new approach. The experienced clinician will be able to read the PDR, drug insert, or medical journal ad and gauge how useful a new drug might be.

However, there are some drugs, not currently in common use, which may prove most valuable. An example is Deaner® (deanol), a drug which is a precursor of acetylcholine. Its administration increases cholinergic transmission in the brain. Another is rubidium, which may prove of value to prevent recurring depression, much as lithium prevents recurring mania. Cyproterone is an antiandrogen which may be useful in reducing sexual drive in patients with sexual impulse behavior disorders.

# CHAPTER 13

# THE PHENOTHIAZINES

THERE are over 2000 phenothiazine drugs. About eighty of them are marketed for psychiatric use. This chapter will go into the phenothiazines in some detail, their effects, and side effects. It should be borne in mind that there are individual differences between the drugs, and that patient response differs to each drug. The patient who does poorly on Thorazine may do well on Stelazine. At present, it is not possible to predict which patient should have which drug or if he should have any drug. If, to use the above example, one knows that Thorazine is the most sedative phenothiazine, while Stelazine is one of the least sedative, a guideline for choice of drug emerges (see Table II).

Most psychiatrists get to know a few phenothiazines well and use them consistently. The non-medical practitioner, who cannot prescribe, may be confronted with a patient taking almost any phenothiazine. However, if he is familiar with what the drug is expected to do and what its side effects may be, he is in a position to offer better service to the patient and give valuable clinical observations to the prescribing doctor.

The phenothiazines are used primarily in treating schizophrenia. They do not "cure" schizophrenia any more than insulin cures diabetes. They control, more or less, the schizophrenic process, including delusional thoughts, hallucinations, illogical thought processes, inability to separate relevant from irrelevant detail, excitement, impulsive behavior, rambling, and tangential speech. They will not mend the personality disorders attendant to a chronic psychosis; the characteristic social withdrawal, inept handling of personal affairs, and crip-

77

*Psychiatric Drugs*

## Table II

### Major Tranquilizers — Dosage and Side Effects

| *Name* | | *Dosage* |
|--------|--|----------|
| Haldol (haloperidol) | | 2 – 80 mg/day* |
| Navane (thiothexene) | | 2 – 60 mg/day |
| Prolixin, Permitil® (fluphenazine) | | 5 – 20 mg/day |
| Prolixin Decanoate® | | 25 – 100 mg/week |
| Prolixin Enanthate® | | 25 – 100 mg/week |
| Stelazine (trifluoperazine) | | 4 – 40 mg/day |
| Quide® (piperacetazine) | | 40 – 160 mg/day |
| Trilafon (perphenazine) | | 4 – 64 mg/day |
| Serentil® (mesoridazine) | | 50 – 400 mg/day |
| Mellaril (thioridazine) | | 25 – 600 mg/day |
| Thorazine (chlorpromazine) | | 25 – 2000 mg/day |

↑ Increasing incidence of extra-pyramidal (parkinsonian) side effects

↓ Increasing incidence of persistent sedation, orthostatic hypotension, allergic responses, seizures

—————
*Mg = milligram, 1/1000 of a gram

pled work life. They may, however, enable the patient to work effectively to acquire these undeveloped or atrophied skills.

The above is a representation of the basic phenothiazine

structure. At this time, it is not clinically important to know the chemical structure of most drugs. However, it is possible that in the future, when the molecular action of these chemicals is known, knowledge of structure will be important in understanding how they work.

$R_1$ and $R_2$ signify chemical groupings which are added on to the phenothiazine nucleus. These groups are known as *radicals*. The unique characteristics of each phenothiazine depends on the nature of the radical groups.

There are three main classes of phenothiazine compounds, based on the type of radical:

1. *Aliphatics* — Milligram for milligram, the aliphatic phenothizines have the least potent antipsychotic effect. They tend to be the most sedative group. The best example is Thorazine (chlorpromazine), the original phenothiazine antipsychotic.
2. *Piperidines* — These types of phenothiazines are less sedating and have less incidence of neurological side effects. The most popular piperidine is Mellaril (thioridazine).
3. *Piperazines* — In this class are the most potent antipsychotics on a dose basis. They tend to be the least sedating, and have the highest incidence of neurological side effects. Stelazine (trifluoperazine) is the most commonly used drug of this type. Prolixin® (fluphenazine) is another popular example of this class.

While phenothiazines differ in potency, as mentioned above, it is important not to attach too much significance to actual milligram dosage. Rather, one should become familiar with the usual dosage range of the major phenothiazines (see Table II). This knowledge can be reassuring to both the patient and the practitioner.

A dosage of 20 mg per day of Stelazine may be adequate for a paranoid schizophrenic patient. An equivalent

dosage of Thorazine would be about 400 mg — twenty
times as much on a weight basis, but with the same antipsychotic effect. Another patient may become anxious if he
is told (usually there is no reason why he should not be
told), that he is taking 1000 mg a day of Thorazine. In
reality, this is one-half of the maximum dosage.

## GROSS BEHAVIORAL EFFECTS OF
## THE PHENOTHIAZINES

The phenothiazines induce a slowing of response to
external stimuli, with decreased initiative, and observable
anxiety. This occurs without the impairment of intellectual ability. With continued administration, tolerance develops to the sedative effect, but not to the antipsychotic
effect. Therefore, a patient who complains of drowsiness
when started on a phenothiazine may be reassured that
this will wear off, usually in a few days. Sometimes, sedation is persistent. The effect of the phenothiazines in reducing reaction to external stimuli may be due to their
effect on the ascending reticular formation (see p. 47).

Another effect on the brain is depression of activity in
the hypothalamus. This may result in disruption of body
temperature regulation by the hypothalamus. In the brain
stem, depression of neural activity causes decreased
peripheral blood pressure. In the spinal cord, there is depression of synaptic reflexes.

The phenothiazines block alpha-adrenergic neurotransmitter activity in the autonomic nervous system. To a
lesser extent, they also block acetylcholine. They probably
have a mild beta-adrenergic stimulating effect. These actions are particularly important when the heart is involved
(see p. 56).

In the skeletal muscles, the phenothiazines induce
muscle relaxation. This makes them of value in some conditions in which there is spastic paralysis — paralysis

induced by disruption of pyramidal tract control (see p. 39).

## Absorption, Fate, and Excretion

The phenothiazines are well absorbed from the gastrointestinal tract. Sixty to 70 percent of a dose is rapidly removed from the portal circulation by the liver, and there is active enterohepatic circulation (see p. 10). The phenothiazines are rapidly distributed to all tissues. They are metabolized mainly by hydroxylation and conjugation with glucuronic acid. There are 168 possible metabolites of Thorazine alone.

Excretion is relatively slow. Although the effects of phenothiazines may be clinically undetectable a few days after administration ceases, various metabolites may be found in the urine six to eighteen months later.

Thorazine is excreted through the kidneys and the gastrointestinal tract, about half in the urine and half in the feces.

The phenothiazines are not addicting. This is important, as many patients fear they will become addicted to medications. A patient going off an antipsychotic medication before he is ready may experience a return of his psychosis. He also may have muscle stiffness and insomnia as the effects of the phenothiazines on his muscles and the CNS subsides. He will not have the psychological and physiological craving for the drug, which marks an addiction. The phenothiazines are not euphoriant; it is no pleasure to take them.

## Preparations

Phenothiazines are available in pill, liquid, suppository, spansule, and injectable form. Mention should be made of the *depot phenothiazines*. In these injectable preparations, the phenothiazine, usually Prolixin, is chemically bonded to a large molecule, either *decanoate* or *enanthate*. The Prolixin Decanoate or Enanthate is injected intramuscularly. Since it is suspended in an oily base, it remains as a deposit rather than being quickly absorbed into the general circulation.

Enzyme action then separates the decanoate or enanthate from the Prolixin molecule, releasing the free phenothiazine. This happens slowly over a one-to-three-week period. Therefore, the patient does not have to take oral medication unless he needs antiparkinsonian medication to relieve side effects. Prolixin Enanthate or Decanoate is particularly useful for long-term schizophrenic patients who are unreliable in taking oral phenothiazines. Research is now in progress on a phenothiazine which can be taken once weekly by mouth.

### General Side Effects

This section is one of the most important for the nonmedical mental health practitioner. In it, most of the side effects which he may observe, and of which the patient may complain, will be discussed along with their physiological mechanisms. It is hoped that familiarity with the material will enable the practitioner to explain these side effects to his patient and gauge their seriousness. He may then convey his observations to the prescribing physician.

These side effects will be discussed in the order in which they are listed in the package insert for Thorazine under the section on adverse reactions. The discussion will be generally applicable to all major tranquilizers. The discussion on neurological side effects will include conditions not mentioned in the Thorazine insert, but which occur more frequently with other antipsychotics.

### Drowsiness

This refers to a state of decreased alertness, with a tendency toward lethargy or sleep. It may be due to the phenothiazines' effect on the reticular activating system, muscular relaxation, and lowered blood pressure. It is not, so far as is known, a cortical effect. Tolerance to drowsiness usually occurs fairly rapidly, but sometimes persists, especially with Thorazine.

### Jaundice

Jaundice is a state of yellow-coloring of the skin and mucous membranes which may be observed in patients with liver damage. It indicates that there has been an escape of bilirubin (see p. 20) from the liver and into the general circulation. The escaped bilirubin enters the skin and the whites of the eyes, imparting a yellow tinge.

Thorazine jaundice is probably due to an allergic reaction. Antibodies to the drug attach to liver cells and, when the drug-antigen reacts with them, the cell membranes are damaged, releasing bilirubin. Since the body must have time to manufacture antibodies, jaundice usually doesn't appear until the second to fourth week of continuous treatment. If the drug is withdrawn, the liver cells will heal, and the jaundice will disappear.

The patient may be given another phenothiazine, such as Mellaril or Stelazine, to which he is not allergic. If possible, it is probably better to switch to a nonphenothiazine antipsychotic, such as Haldol or Navane. Thorazine jaundice is rarely seen these days, having been much more common in the early days of the use of the drug. Its relative rarity now may be due to refinements of the manufacturing process.

## Hematological Disorders

It is somewhat ironic that most neurological side effects, while spectacular and alarming, are not particularly dangerous and are easily treated. But a relatively common physical symptom, a sore throat, may herald a potentially deadly drug reaction, a blood dyscrasia. The blood dyscrasias, agranulocytosis, eosinophilia, leukopenia, hemolytic anemia, thrombocytopenic purpura and pancytopenia have all been discussed above (see pp. 64-66).

The appearance of sore throat, fever, gum sores, bruises, or general severe fatigue may be danger signs in a patient taking phenothiazines. Immediate medical attention is necessary including appropriate laboratory tests.

As with jaundice, blood dyscrasias are probably allergenic in origin. They usually occur four to ten weeks after beginning therapy but may occur at any time. For this reason, semiannual blood counts are advisable on all patients taking chronic phenothiazines.

## Cardiovascular Side Effects

### Hypotensive Reactions

*Orthostatic,* or *postural* hypotension means that when the patient moves from a recumbent to a standing position, his blood pressure falls. This may result in a feeling of dizziness, unsteadiness, or even fainting, due to a temporarily inadequate supply of blood to the brain. The phenothiazines may cause this by interfering with the body's normal compensatory mechanisms for maintaining stable blood pressure when moving into an upright position.

Compensatory mechanisms include increased heart rate, constriction of blood vessels, and increased strength of heart contractions. Interference with these mechanisms is due to the phenothiazine's effect on the brain stem, where vascular reflexes are controlled, and the adrenergic effects on the heart and large blood vessels.

It is possible, though very uncommon, for an injected phenothiazine to cause a life-threatening drop in blood pressure. The pressure may fall so low that the patient goes into *shock,* that state in which there is inadequate circulation, therefore, inadequate oxygenation, which leads to abnormal metabolism in vital organs, the brain, heart and kidneys. If shock is not controlled in time, irreversible tissue damage may occur, leading to death.

In connection with this, it is important for the practitioner to understand the *reversed epinephrine effect* of the phenothiazines. Knowledge of this mechanism could conceivably be lifesaving.

As discussed above, the phenothiazines are alpha-adrenergic blockers. They are also beta-adrenergic stimulators, producing vasodilatation. There are both alpha- and beta-adrenergic receptors on blood vessels. The alpha-receptors cause constriction. The beta-receptors cause dilatation (see p. 29).

Epinephrine, or *adrenalin,* acts at both alpha- and beta-receptors. When the alpha-adrenergic receptors are blocked by a phenothiazine, epinephrine apparently reaches mainly the beta-receptors, resulting in an epinephrine-induced dilatation of blood vessels. This causes a decrease in the effective blood volume, since the same volume of blood is now in a larger space. This leads to a further lowering of an already low blood pressure.

Therefore, in treating phenothiazine-induced shock, epinephrine should *not* be used. Instead, an agent which acts only on the alpha-adrenergic receptors, such as Levophed®, or Neo-Synephrine®, is employed. These drugs will compete with the phenothiazine for the alpha-adrenergic sites and cause constriction of the blood vessels and stronger heart contractions with a resultant rise in blood pressure.

Most cases of phenothiazine shock can be treated simply by placing the patient in a supine position (on his back), raising his legs and, if necessary, administering intravenous fluids and oxygen. However, if it is necessary to increase blood pressure by use of a drug, it is vital to know the above information.

Since epinephrine is often one of the first drugs resorted to in treating shock, the attending physician must be aware of the reversed epinephrine effect. If he is not aware of it (and no physician knows everything), a word from the non-medical practitioner may not only be appreciated but lifesaving.

### EKG Changes

The phenothiazines are depressants of cardiac muscle excitability. In rare instances, this can mean a critical reduction in strength of cardiac contractions. If a patient's heart muscle is already weakened because of coronary artery disease or other illness, a phenothiazine could further weaken the heart to the point of causing heart failure. Most people have an adequate *cardiac reserve* so that this action of the phenothiazines is negligible. However, phenothiazines must be used cautiously and in minimum dosage with patients who have a history of cardiac disease.

Even in normal individuals, the cardiac-depressant action of the phenothiazines may result in changes in the electrocardiogram. The EKG is basically a recording of electrical activity accompanying muscle contraction in the heart. Minor changes in the EKG are often seen in patients taking phenothiazines.

## Neurological Side Effects

The most widely accepted theory of how the phenothiazines and other antipsychotic drugs work is that they block dopamine neurotransmission in the brain. Where this action occurs in order to result in an antipsychotic effect is not definitely known. Probably, structures in the limbic system and adjacent areas and the reticular activating system are important in antipsychotic action. Blockade of noradrenergic neurons and/or dopaminergic neurons is another possible mechanism.

However, blockade of known dopaminergic tracts explains some common undesirable side effects of the phenothiazines. As discussed earlier (Chapter 7), there are dopaminergic tracts in the extrapyramidal structures, especially the caudate nucleus. When the phenothiazines block tracts in these structures, a chemically induced Parkinson's disease results. The patient displays a masklike face, shuffling gait, cogwheel rigidity of his arms, and sometimes drools uncontrollably (see Fig. 24).

The extrapyramidal system contains tracts which utilize acetylcholine as the main neurotransmitter. These cholinergic tracts and the dopaminergic tracts act in balance with each other. For this reason, a drug which is anticholinergic, when given to a parkinsonian patient, partially restores the balance and relieves at least some symptoms. A patient on the phenothiazines who has parkinsonian side effects is often treated with an antiparkinsonian drug, such as Cogentin, Artane, Tremin® or Kemedrin®. These drugs exert an anticholinergic effect in the brain. The antihistaminic medication Benadryl, is also sometimes used. These drugs also relieve other neurological side effects to be discussed below.

### Motor Restlessness

This is a neurological side effect which may be mistaken for a manifestation of the patient's psychiatric condition.

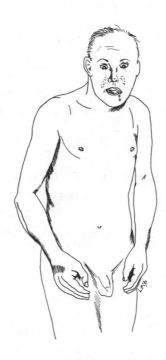

PHENOTHIAZINE SIDE EFFECT
PATIENT WITH CHEMICALLY INDUCED PARKINSON'S DISEASE

Figure 24.

The technical name for it is *akathisia*. The patient desires to be in continuous motion. He cannot sit still and may pace. He feels anxious. When he is sitting, his legs are often in motion and he displays stepping movements or swinging of the lower legs. Obviously this behavior may be mistaken for manifestations of anxiety and agitation. The phenothiazines may then be increased, thereby aggravating or at least not lessening the akathisia. As with parkinsonian side effects, akathisia may be relieved by the use of Cogentin, or Artane. Minor tranquilizers, such as Valium, or antihistamine medications may be used.

## *Akinesia*

In contrast to motor restlessness, patients on phenothiazine may develop an extrapyramidal side effect characterized by reduced spontaneity, diminished speech, infrequent gestures, and apparent apathy. It can be confused with depression or psychosis. The patient has difficulty in initiating his usual activities. A diagnostic point is that the reduced spontaneity applies to all activities, not just those about which there may be some emotional conflict. This syndrome, too, may be treated with antiparkinsonian drugs.

## **The Dystonias**

Dystonia is a general term indicating loss of normal muscular tone. If the muscle tone of a particular group of muscles is either exaggerated or abnormally reduced, abnormal positions of the respective body parts results. Muscle groups are balanced in their actions. In the legs and arms, there are *flexor groups*, which bend, and *extensor groups*, which straighten. If one group is paralyzed or weakened, the other will act alone, and the limb will assume an abnormal position.

There are continuous impulses flowing from the brain down the pyramidal tracts and influenced by the extrapyramidal system. These impulses flow to the muscles, maintaining a continuous tone: In the normal individual, muscles are never completely relaxed. Dystonias are probably the result of the effects of the phenothiazines on the cranial outflow to the muscles, via the pyramidal and extrapyramidal systems. Phenothiazine interference with adrenergic transmission causes muscular imbalance and spasm of various muscle groups resulting in characteristic clinical pictures. Dystonias occur most frequently in young male patients. These side effects are particularly frightening to the patient, who may experience them as paralyses or even seizures. They may also be alarming to the uninformed therapist. In reality, they are almost never in themselves dangerous and are easily treated with antiparkinsonian drugs, usually given by injection for rapid effect. They are *not* contraindications to the continued use of the drug. Of course, dosage may be reduced and/or regular use of antiparkinsonian drugs may

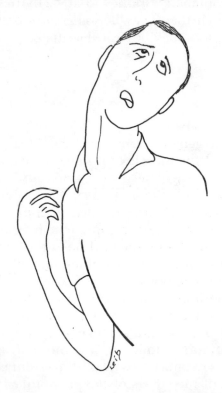

## DYSTONIAS

Figure 25.

be instituted.

The following are descriptions of the major dystonias:

*Opisthotonus* - The patient assumes a position in which the head and heels bend backwards; the midsection bows forward. This may be due to major interference with the pyramidal and extrapyramidal outflow, resulting in the more powerful muscle groups overcoming the weaker. The body assumes a position resulting from this muscular imbalance.

*Oculogyric Crisis* - This is a very distressing side effect in which a spasm of the eye muscles causes fixed, painful upward gaze. The patient cannot control his eye movements. It usually occurs one to two days after starting on a phenothiazine, as do most dystonias (see Fig. 25).

*Torticollis* - In this dystonia there is an imbalance of the "strap" muscles of the neck. The head is involuntarily turned to one side. There may also be an associated spasm of the mouth and tongue muscles resulting in tongue protrusion and difficulty in talking and swallowing.

When the above reactions occur, the patient may be understandably reluctant to continue taking his medication. However, he can be reassured that they are not serious conditions and usually do not recur. They are not allergies, although many patients will report them as such. (One often hears, "I'm allergic to the phenothiazines," from a patient who has been through a dystonic reaction.)

### Tremor

Tremor is defined as alternating movements caused by the contraction of opposing muscle groups. It may occur at any time during course of treatment with many psychotropic drugs. It should be distinguished from the tremor of anxiety. The patient will often feel calm despite the tremor.

## Tardive Dyskinesia

This is the most serious of the neurological side effects induced by antipsychotic medications. Unlike the dystonias, tardive dyskinesia may be associated with actual brain-tissue damage causing a permanent condition.

Tardive dyskinesia is characterized by involuntary abnormal mouth or tongue movements which resemble facial tics. The earliest sign is often slight "wormlike" twitching movements of the tongue, best seen when the patient opens his mouth with the tongue in a relaxed position. There may be mild mouthing or chewing movements. This may progress to involuntary tongue protrusion with thrusting, rolling, "flycatching" tongue motions. The patient may develop slow, writhing, purposeless movements in his arms and legs. Rarely, a to-and-fro rocking motion is present.

Tardive dyskinesia usually occurs in patients who have taken antipsychotic medication for years. Rarely, it occurs after a few months or weeks of treatment. Women patients older than age fifty comprise the highest percentage of cases, but it has been seen in all age groups. Oddly, the patient himself often is not particularly troubled by the condition, distressing as it appears to family and therapist.

The neurophysiology of tardive dyskinesia is especially important as it sheds some light on the action of psychotropic drugs.

The antipsychotics are dopamine blockers. It is postulated that when dopamine blockade occurs over a long period, the nervous system begins to respond in several ways. The dopamine receptors become ultrasensitive. Since they are not getting the usual amount of dopamine necessary to fire them, they become sensitive to lesser amounts, those which get past the blockading antipsychotic drug.

Next, the dopamine receptors may increase in number.

Eventually, there may be irreversible damage to the synaptic membranes of dopaminergic neurons. This state of affairs results in certain dopamine tracts becoming very sensitive, with many receptors firing in an abnormal manner. This, in turn, produces the abnormal movements discussed above.

At present, there is no cure for tardive dyskinesia. If it is detected early enough, the antipsychotic medication may be stopped, and the dopamine receptors will return to normal. Periodic observation of a patient's tongue, to look for telltale twitching movements is the simplest precaution. Some patients can safely take "drug holidays": They do not take their antipsychotic medications one or two days a week. On these drug holidays the tardive dyskinesia may become apparent, as it is masked by the presence of the very drug that causes it.

The employment of minimal dosage is another preventative, as well as being a good rule for any medication.

At present, the treatment for tardive dyskinesia is unsatisfactory. The antiparkinsonian drugs have no effect. Reserpine, which reduces the dopamine content of the brain, may be used. Deanol, an acetylcholine precursor, has been tried successfully but is not yet an established treatment.

However, the dopamine-blocking antipsychotics, which cause the disease in the first place, may be used to treat it. Since these drugs block dopamine receptors, they reduce abnormal dopamine tract activity. Unfortunately, this can lead to a worsening of the condition, which is concealed while the patient is taking the antipsychotic, and becomes manifest when the drug is stopped.

## Adverse Behavioral Effects

For reasons which are not clear, a rare patient may react to an antipsychotic drug by going into a psychotic state.

This side effect is hard to recognize.

## Cerebral Edema

Edema is due to a passage of fluid out of tissue and vessels and into the surrounding space. The phenothiazines probably alter membrane permeability and, in susceptible individuals, may cause fluid to accumulate in the brain. This is a rare, potentially fatal condition which the non-medical practitioner would not be expected to diagnose. Should it occur, it would be obvious that the patient was gravely ill with symptoms such as vomiting, fever, coma, respiratory difficulty, and rapid heart.

## Seizures

The phenothiazines lower the *seizure threshold* in patients who have epilepsy. This means that a patient who is seizure prone must be treated with the lowest possible dose. He may also need to be covered with an antiseizure medication, such as Dilantin. The antipsychotics differ in their seizure-promoting properties (see Table II). The mechanism of this effect is not known. It may be due to the phenothiazines lowering the amount of a neurotransmitter called *Gamma Amino Butyric Acid* (GABA) in the brain. Deficiency of GABA has been described in the cortex of epileptics.

## Allergic Reactions

As is the case with most foreign substances, allergies can develop with the phenothiazines (see Chapter 11). The drug becomes attached to plasma proteins and becomes antigenic. The drug-protein antigen stimulates antibody formation. The antibodies attach to various body organs, and the stage is set for an allergic reaction the next time the drug is given.

Skin allergies are frequent allergic manifestations caused by the phenothiazines. The following types of skin reactions occur:

### Rash

This is a general term referring to an abnormal appearance of the skin, usually an area of redness or tiny red to purple dots, *petechiae*, which are caused either by dilatation of skin capillaries or bleeding into the skin. If bleeding is extensive, a blotchy rash called purpura develops. This may be due to a severe allergic reaction, but the possibility of infection should be considered.

### Photosensitivity

In this condition, the circulating phenothiazine-protein passes through capillaries in the skin. When exposed to sunlight, a reaction occurs which is essentially a severe sunburn. (This may also be due to phenothiazine interference with melanin production [see section on endocrinology].) This is not an allergic reaction, because antibody production is not essential to its occurrence.

In fact, it is so common that patients taking phenothiazines, especially Thorazine, must be routinely cautioned against too much sun exposure. Some patients need a sunscreening preparation, such as Uvral®, during the summer months. For some reason, this reaction does not occur with Mellaril, making it the drug of choice for patients who cannot avoid a lot of outdoor activity.

### Urticaria

An urticaria is a hive, an itchy, elevated patch of skin, which is either redder or paler than the surrounding skin.

It is a true allergic reaction, and may occur at the site of an injection or be generalized over the entire body.

### Exfoliative Dermatitis

This severe allergic reaction is characterized by scaling and peeling of the skin along with itching, fever, and malaise. It may be a drug reaction to the phenothiazines (or other drug), but it may also be a sign of a more serious underlying condition, such as leukemia or malignant tumor. Any patient displaying such a severe reaction deserves a complete medical workup.

### Anaphylaxis

Though very uncommon, this severe allergic reaction can occur with the phenothiazines. It is characterized by edema of the larynx and spasm of the bronchi (air tubes), interfering with respiration. Vascular collapse occurs with a low blood pressure and massive vasodilatation. It almost always happens after an injection, rather than oral administration. The treatment includes placing the patient in *shock position*, the body supine with the legs a little raised, maintenance of an open airway, and oxygen administration. Drugs employed include epinephrine (1 cc of a 1:1000 solution I.M. or I.V.), antihistamines, (Benadryl 50 to 150 mg I.M.), and sometimes steroids (see Chapter 11 for a discussion of the allergic mechanisms of anaphylaxis).

## Endocrine Disorders

As outlined in Chapter 7, hormonal regulation is dependent on normal function of the pituitary gland and the hypothalamus. The neurotransmitter control of the pituitary by the hypothalamus involves dopaminergic tracts.

Since the antipsychotics interfere with dopamine transmission, endocrine disturbances can occur in patients
taking these drugs.

## Lactation

Lactation means secretion of milk from the breast. It is
stimulated by the hormone *prolactin*. Prolactin is released
from the anterior pituitary. Its release is prevented by a
prolactin inhibiting factor from the hypothalamus. This
factor may be blocked by a phenothiazine, resulting in
prolactin release, breast enlargement, and lactation. This
can be an alarming side effect, which the patient may not
associate with the drug. The uninformed therapist might
pass off such a complaint as delusional.

## Amenorrhea

Amenorrhea is the cessation of the menstrual cycle.
Menstrual abnormalities can occur in women taking antipsychotics, as the drug may interfere with the shifting
hormonal balance of the normal cycle. In combination
with the side effect of lactation, the patient (and therapist),
may believe she is pregnant. These effects can be reduced
or eliminated by adjustment of dosage, or by changing to
another medication. (Another neuroendocrine effect usually observed in women is an increased desire for sexual
activity.)

## Hyperglycemia, Hypoglycemia, Glucosuria

These terms refer respectively to elevated blood sugar,
low blood sugar, and sugar in the urine. Blood sugar level
is controlled by insulin secreted by specialized cells in the
pancreas. Phenothiazines may affect insulin secretion by
direct action on these cells. A patient who is a borderline

diabetic might become diabetic when on a phenothiazine.

## Autonomic Reactions

Almost all antipsychotic drugs are anticholinergic (see Chapter 5). Some drugs are much more so than others, and this may be a determining factor in drug choice and dosage. As discussed above, *anticholinergic* refers to blockage of access of acetylcholine to its receptor sites in the parasympathetic autonomic nervous system or the brain. An understanding of this mechanism readily explains the following effects.

### Dry Mouth

The parasympathetic nerves to the salivary glands are blocked, reducing saliva secretion. This may be partially compensated by drinking frequently or chewing gum. The effect usually wears off as the patient continues taking the drug.

### Constipation

Parasympathetic impulses to the intestines stimulate motion of the gut. If they are blocked, reduced gut motion and constipation results. This effect will usually disappear with time. If it continues, the use of bulk foods, such as bran, may be indicated. Laxatives over long periods are not advisable, since they may result in reduced muscular tone in the intestines and loss of sodium and potassium, chemicals important in body functioning.

### Adynamic Ileus

This is complete paralysis of the intestines characterized by bloating of the abdomen, vomiting, and pain. It is an extreme anticholinergic effect and is rare during treatment with phenothiazines. It is most likely to occur with overdosage.

### Urinary Retention

Bladder paralysis may occur as a result of anticholinergic action on the nerves supplying the bladder wall muscles. The patient may report a lessening of the force of his urinary stream. If the patient has preexisting prostate disease already interfering with urine flow, inability to expel urine may occur. In extreme cases, this may require catheterization to relieve urine buildup in the bladder.

### Impotence

This is also an anticholinergic effect, most commonly encountered with Mellaril. The patient may be unable to have an erection, or may not ejaculate. Sometimes the patient may experience orgasm but without ejaculation. It is a distressing side effect and the patient should be warned in advance, or he may otherwise not associate it with the drug.

### Miosis

This refers to constriction of the pupil, which usually occurs with overdosage.

### Mydriasis

This is the term for enlargement of the pupil, a common anticholinergic effect. It is really the result of the unopposed action of the sympathetic nerves on the pupil. As discussed in Chapter 10, it may precipitate an attack of glaucoma.

### Skin Pigmentation

In patients who take the phenothiazines over a period of

years, skin pigmentation may be observed. This can range from a darkening of exposed skin areas to an actual grayish purple color. This effect is generally seen in patients who have been hospitalized for years. The mechanism is unknown. One theory is that the antipsychotics affect secretion of the MSH from the middle lobe of the pituitary (see Chapter 8). Increased MSH would result in more secretion of melanin, darkening the skin. A melanin-like compound, possibly a complex of the phenothiazine with melanin, has been found in the dermis in such patients. Another theory is that attachment of the drug to cell membranes affects their color. This effect may fade if the drug is discontinued.

### Ocular Changes

Tiny granules have been observed in the corneas and lenses of patients taking antipsychotics in large doses over long periods, especially Thorazine. These granules, the nature of which is unknown, do not interfere with vision, but are permanent. They most often develop in patients taking 500 mg or more per day of Thorazine continuously for six months. More seriously, darkening of the retina due to deposit of a pigment has been seen in some patients, especially those taking Mellaril in doses over 1000 mg a day for months. This results in a decrease in night visual acuity. Patients on the antipsychotics should have regular or yearly eye checkups.

### Other Side Effects

Since the phenothiazines affect the temperature-regulation centers in the hypothalamus, abnormalities of body temperature may occur. Hypothalamic centers controlling appetite may also be affected, resulting in increased appetite and weight gain.

The phenothiazines reduce nausea and vomiting and are sometimes medically employed for that purpose. Curiously, however, many patients taking them complain of nausea. The mechanism for this is not clear but may be due to local irritation of stomach tissue by the drugs themselves. This can be relieved by the simultaneous administration of an antacid such as Maalox®.

Phenothiazines also increase the effects, or *potentiate,* of other drugs which affect the CNS, such as analgesics, sedatives, and alcohol.

### Death

The package insert on Thorazine mentions ". . . occasional reports of sudden death in patients receiving phenothiazines," but comfortingly continues, "There is not sufficient evidence to establish a relationship between such deaths and the administration of phenothiazines." The phenothiazines and other antipsychotics affect the heart, they affect the autonomic nervous system, and they affect the hypothalamic-adrenal axis (a crucial mechanism of response to stress). In one study, a very high death rate was observed in surgical patients who had been on phenothiazines.

The point of the above is not to argue against the use of these valuable drugs, but that they should be used with caution. A patient on phenothiazines who must undergo surgery should have prescribed phenothiazines reduced to a minimum or discontinued, if possible. The surgeon and anesthetist should be informed of the type, dose, and duration of administration.

### Other Antipsychotics

The terms *phenothiazines* and *antipsychotics* are used almost interchangeably in the above discussion. The clinician should be aware that there are several groups of nonphenothiazine antipsychotics. They seem to have all the side effects of the phenothiazines and are useful for the same conditions. For reasons which are unknown, some patients will do better on a nonphenothiazine antipsychotic. Patients allergic to a phenothiazine will probably not be allergic to a chemically different compound. The various groups and representative examples follow. It should be remembered that the data presented above on the phenothiazines generally applies to nonphenothiazines.

### Butyrophenones

This group is generally less sedative than the phenothiazines. A representative type is Haldol. It has been found to be particularly useful in elderly patients. When used with younger patients, there is a high incidence of dystonias which must be managed with antiparkinsonian drugs.

### Thioxanthenes

This antipsychotic is exemplified by Navane, a drug which is claimed to have some antidepressant effect.

### Dihydroindolone

The only marketed example of this chemical group is Moban. This drug is claimed to have an alerting affect on chronic, apathetic schizophrenics. The site of action is stated to be the ascending reticular formation, a structure mediating alertness and screening of environmental data (see p. 47). The side effects are similar to those of the other antipsychotics.

## Loxapine Succinate

This is the only representative of a class of antipsychotics which have a tricyclic structure somewhat similar to that of an important group of antidepressant drugs (see Chapter 14). The trade name is Loxitane®. In animal studies, the sites of action appear to be the midbrain and the reticular formation. The drug is claimed to be useful for symptoms of irritability and hostility in schizophrenics, as well as causing the usual improvement in thought disorder and hallucinations characteristic of psychotic states.

# ANTIDEPRESSANTS

THIS chapter will cover the medications used in the treatment of depression.

It has been repeatedly observed that patients are generally more cooperative in taking antidepressant than antipsychotic drugs, even though the drugs share many unpleasant side effects. This is probably because depression feels worse than schizophrenia. The chronic schizophrenic's symptoms are often more troublesome to his family and associates than to himself.

The depressed patient, on the other hand, feels terrible. He experiences profound, unrealistic, but no less real feelings of hopelessness and despair. He sees the world "through a glass darkly." Life has no savor. The most sought-after success brings no joy; unhappy events may not call forth appropriate sadness. Physical symptoms occur, with sluggishness, fatigue, constipation, dry mouth, loss of appetite, and decreased libido as common complaints.

Depressions are generally divided into two main types: *reactive* and *endogenous*. Antidepressant drugs are mainly useful in the latter category.

Endogenous depressions may have no clear precipitant: A tendency to experience depression seems inherent in the personality of the affected individual. When genuinely depressing events have occurred, the ensuing depression is abnormally prolonged and may be the deepening of a preexisting depressive mood. The endogenously depressed patient suffers impairment of his ability to cope. He may be immobilized. Nothing alleviates the depression, even momentarily. He may be preoccupied with feelings of worthlessness and guilt. In extreme cases, delusions based on these feelings may occur. Suicide may terminate a depression. Suicidal risk must be monitored throughout the course of this disease.

Reactive depressions have a clear precipitant and are usually self-limiting. The patient's coping techniques remain intact and are at least somewhat effective in alleviating his unhappiness. Depressions follow a consistent course. They begin, are present from three months to a year, and they remit. A patient can be confidently reassured that his depression will eventually end. Some clinicians feel that the antidepressants accelerate the course of the disease, hastening normal remission. On the other hand, some feel that there are depressive individuals for whom the antidepressants normalize a genetic tendency to neurohumeral imbalance. These patients may take antidepressants for many years, even for their entire lifetime.

Antidepressant medications must be distinguished from stimulants. Stimulants cause feelings of euphoria; antidepressants do not. Antidepressants relieve depression but do not make the patient feel "happy," as the stimulants do.

There are two main groups of antidepressants, the *tricyclics,* and the *monoamine oxidase inhibitors* (MAOI's). The tricyclics are more widely used and will be considered first.

The following are the structural formulas for Tofranil and Elavil, two widely used tricyclics. It may be noted that their structures resemble the basic phenothiazine structure. Actually, the phenothiazines and the tricyclics share many pharmacologic properties. With regard to side effects, both are anticholinergic. Tricyclics, however, are more dangerous to the heart, and, if taken in overdose or by susceptible individuals, have more serious side effects in the brain itself.

TOFRANIL                    ELAVIL

## General Effects of the Tricyclics

### *Central Nervous System*

Tricyclics cause a general decrease in total electrical activity in the brain, as measured by the electroencephalogram (EEG). In this respect, they resemble the effects of drugs which block cholinergic transmission. There is relief of depressive feelings. Rarely, normal doses may cause delirium with excitement and hallucinations.

### *Autonomic Nervous System*

In the autonomic nervous system, the action of acetylcholine blockade is prominent, with dry mouth, blurred vision, constipation, and urinary retention as possible effects. In some patients, increased sweating may occur (see Table III).

### *Cardiovascular System*

The tricyclics decrease cardiac reflexes, lowering blood pressure and inducing orthostatic hypotension (see p. 84).

### Table III

### Anticholinergic and Sedative Properties of Tricyclic Antidepressants

*Anticholinergic Effects of Tricyclics*

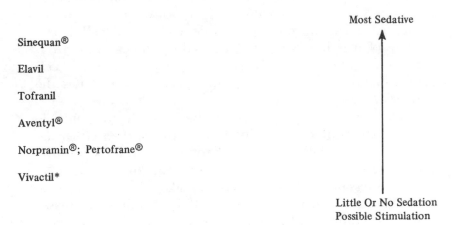

Most Anticholinergic

Elavil

Tofranil

Aventyl®; Sinequan®; Adapin®

Norpramin®; Pertofrane®

Increasing anticholinergic effects — dry mouth, blurred vision, constipation, etc.

Least Anticholinergic

*Sedative Effects of Tricyclics*

Most Sedative

Sinequan®

Elavil

Tofranil

Aventyl®

Norpramin®; Pertofrane®

Vivactil*

Little Or No Sedation
Possible Stimulation

---

*This drug is stimulant in many patients, sometimes causing agitation and restlessness.

They may also weaken heart action to the point of precipitating heart failure, in patients with preexisting cardiac disease. The heart tends to beat faster due to blockade of the vagus nerve.

## Mechanism of Action

As with other psychotropic drugs, the mechanism of action is not known precisely. However, there is a fairly coherent theory about the action of the tricyclics based on a theory of the biochemical roots of depression.

As discussed elsewhere (see p. 33), the brain's synapses utilize a variety of neurotransmitters; acetylcholine, dopamine, norepinephrine, and serotonin. As is known and well demonstrated by such disorders as Parkinson's disease, these neurotransmitters must be in balance with each other for healthy functioning. It is possible that depression may be due to increased cholinergic transmission and a deficit of catecholamine transmitter action (norepinephrine, dopamine, and serotonin).

In a catecholamine transmitter nerve ending, the transmitter is synthesized and stored in a submicroscopic storage granule. When the nerve is stimulated, the transmitter is released from the granule to the nerve cell, where some of it is immediately destroyed by the enzyme MAO. Some of the transmitter passes through the nerve cell membrane, crosses the synaptic space, and activates the receptor.

The receptor may be on another nerve cell, a muscle cell, a sweat gland, etc. The transmitter is then either destroyed by further enzymatic action or taken back into the cell from which it was released (see Fig. 26). The tricyclic antidepressants act to prevent uptake of catecholamine transmitters into nerve endings. This effectively increases the concentration of norepinephrine, dopamine and serotonin at their receptor sites.

It is theorized that the increased concentration of these transmitters, acting at unknown sites in the brain, relieves depression, either by increasing catecholamine transmitter activity or restoring the balance when there is excessive cholinergic transmission. The suspected sites are the

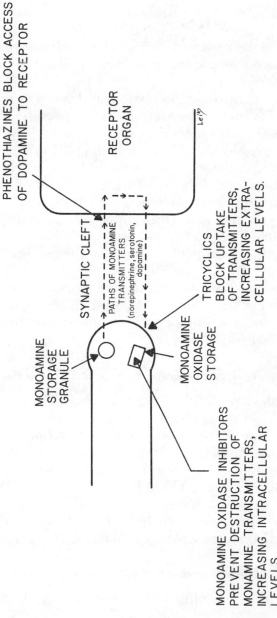

PHENOTHIAZINES BLOCK ACCESS OF DOPAMINE TO RECEPTOR

RECEPTOR ORGAN

SYNAPTIC CLEFT

PATHS OF MONOAMINE TRANSMITTERS (norepinephrine, serotonin, dopamine)

TRICYCLICS BLOCK UPTAKE OF TRANSMITTERS, INCREASING EXTRA-CELLULAR LEVELS.

MONOAMINE STORAGE GRANULE

MONOAMINE OXIDASE STORAGE

MONOAMINE OXIDASE INHIBITORS PREVENT DESTRUCTION OF MONAMINE TRANSMITTERS, INCREASING INTRACELLULAR LEVELS.

NERVE ENDING & RECEPTOR SHOWING NEUROTRANSMITTERS AND SITES OF ACTIONS OF VARIOUS DRUG TYPES

Figure 26.

reticular formation and the amygdalae in the midbrain (see p. 46). The midbrain contains structures which apparently mediate "reward" behavior. The receptors in these areas may be mainly noradrenergic, utilizing norepinephrine and dopamine. Areas of the hypothalamus also may be involved.

It should be pointed out, however, that this theory of the mechanism of action of the tricyclics is not proven. There are studies with experimental evidence that at least one tricyclic does *not* block uptake of norepinephrine. There is also evidence that the tricyclics actually block adrenergic receptors. The standard theory of tricyclic mechanism ignores the anticholinergic action of the tricyclics in the brain, an effect which is of great importance in toxic reactions (see below).

The fact is that theories of action of all the psychotropic drugs are based on our present incomplete knowledge of normal brain function, especially with respect to neurotransmitters. The theories are useful models, but, will probably be proven wrong or, at best, only approximately correct. Learn them anyway.

### Absorption, Distribution, Fate, and Excretion

The tricyclics are rapidly absorbed from the intestinal tract, strongly bound to plasma proteins, and very actively metabolized. One of the major metabolic actions is the removal of methyl ($CH_3$) groups. The demethylated form of Tofranil is marketed as Norpramin and Pertofrane and the demethylated form of Elavil is sold as Aventyl. About one third of the tricyclics are excreted through the G.I. tract and the other two-thirds through the kidneys. There is also an active enterohepatic circulation (see p. 10).

### Dosage and Administration

It is a curious, but clinically important, fact that the

antidepressants take several days to several weeks to work. The patient may feel nothing but the side effects for weeks after beginning the drug. Some patients may respond to as little as 25 mg per day of a tricyclic. Others may need as much as 300 mg per day. A patient who is deriving no benefit from a dose of 200 mg per day may respond well to 250 mg.

Doses are administered in pill form, occasionally in liquid concentrates, and a few in injectibles. It takes knowledge, skill and patience for the clinician to use these drugs properly. The patient, too, must be cooperative during the early phase of treatment. An area under development, which may alleviate this problem, is the measurement of plasma concentration of the tricyclics and other drugs. Eventually, it should be possible routinely to take a blood sample and ascertain the plasma level of psychotropic drugs. Measurement of plasma concentrations may then be correlated with clinical response. There seems to be a range of concentration at which the best clinical response is obtained. Below this concentration and, surprisingly, above it, response is suboptimal. (It should be remembered that concentration in the plasma does not necessarily reflect concentration in the brain.)

## SIDE EFFECTS

### Anticholinergic Side Effects

Tricyclics are chemically similar to the phenothiazines and share many side effects with them. The potential side effects and their mechanisms are essentially the same for allergic reactions, endocrine effects, and most cardiovascular and anticholinergic symptoms. However, the anticholinergic side effects seem to be more pronounced with the tricyclics — patients especially complain of dry mouth and constipation. These side effects may be treated with medications which mimic or enhance the action of acetyl-choline.

One such drug is Urecholine® (bethanecol chloride), a drug which acts like acetylcholine at parasympathetic nerve endings in the bladder, intestines and salivary glands. Twenty-five mg of this drug three times a day may relieve the dry mouth, the constipation, and difficult urination some patients experience with the tricyclics.

## Cardiovascular Side Effects

### Hypertension and Hypotension

The tricyclics may produce low blood pressure (hypotension) by inhibiting the reflexes which normally maintain adequate blood pressure as the body changes position. Hypertension may occur through the increase in circulating catecholamines, such as norepinephrine, produced by the tricyclics' inhibition of catecholamine uptake from peripheral nerve endings. This may be a potentially serious side effect if the patient is already hypertensive (has high blood pressure).

A drug sometimes used in treating hypertension, Ismelin® (guanethedine), acts as a false neurotransmitter. It must be taken up into neuronal endings to work. If a patient is taking a tricyclic, the uptake of guanethedine will be inhibited and the treatment will be correspondingly ineffective. This is an example of drug interactions, an area so complex that a detailed treatment is beyond the scope of this book. The non-medical practitioner should be aware that interactions between drugs do occur, and that these interactions can be harmful.

### Myocardial Infarction

Myocardial infarction, commonly called *heart attack,*

refers to the damage to heart muscle which occurs when there is inadequate blood supply to an area of the heart itself. Heart tissue is supplied by a system of vessels called coronary arteries, so an infarct is also a *coronary*.

Myocardial infarctions may be caused by many factors; there are several related to the effects of the tricyclics. They cause anticholinergic blockade of the vagus nerve and, by increasing catecholamines, boost sympathetic activity. This may result in an abnormally rapid heart rate. An overactive heart, whose coronary vessels may be only marginally supplying its tissue, is ripe for a myocardial infarction. This can also happen if there is tricyclic-induced hypotension or disturbance of the heart's regular rhythm.

### Arrhythmias and Heart Block

Disturbance in the regular beat of the heart may occur because of tricyclic effect on the heart's conduction system (see p. 56).

Impulses from the atria to the ventricles may be blocked. The autonomic action of the drugs may also cause irregularity of rhythm. In cases of overdosage, severe irregularities may lead to a cardiac arrest. In low dosage, the tricyclic effect is mainly to block the vagus nerve. In higher dosage, it seems to affect the heart tissue as well. This is probably related to tricyclic-induced excesses of catecholamines. Catecholamines are beta-adrenergic stimulators. Beta-adrenergic receptors in the heart stimulate increased rate and increased sensitivity of cardiac tissue (see p. 29). Therefore, in cases of tricyclic overdosage, a beta-adrenergic blocking agent, such as Inderal® (propanolol) may be used in the treatment of cardiac complications.

The tricyclics must be used with caution in patients with heart disease. There seem to be varying degrees of cardiotoxicity associated with different tricyclics. Tofranil and Elavil are mentioned fairly frequently in the literature on cardiac complications. On the other hand, little or no cardiac toxic effects are reported for Sinequan; it is often used in older patients for this reason.

Tricyclic poisoning in children has become a serious problem. There have been adverse effects observed in newborns whose mothers took Tofranil in pregnancy. Patients with children should be cautioned to keep their antidepressants and other drugs in childproof containers, out of reach. The child himself may be the patient, as Tofranil has been used successfully in the treatment of bed-wetting (enuresis), and some behavior disorders of childhood, such as hyperactivity and school phobias.

### Central Nervous System Effects

A major difference between the tricyclics and the phenothiazines is that the tricyclics rarely produce extrapyramidal side effects. While some patients may have a mild tremor, there are no alarming dystonias.

However, there are serious neurological side effects associated with tricyclic use. Most of these may be explained by the drugs' actions as blockers of cholinergic transmission.

One of the most serious of these effects is the activation or reactivation of latent psychosis. There have been cases of stable schizophrenic patients who, placed on a tricyclic, became delusional again. If one considers the dopamine hypothesis of schizophrenia, a possible mechanism emerges. Schizophrenia may be associated with excess or abnormal dopamine transmission. Dopamine tracts may act in balance with cholinergic tracts. If the tricyclics block acetylcholine transmission, this balance may be upset. Moreover, such cholinergic blockade would, in effect, create an excess of dopamine transmission. Another possibility is that blockage of reuptake of catecholamines produces increased dopamine transmission.

Consideration of the effects of a large overdose of a tricyclic provides a model for review of parasympathetic activity, as well as an important clinical situation which the therapist may face.

The patient who takes an overdose of a tricyclic blocks most of the body's acetylcholine transmission. It is similar to taking a large amount of atropine, the classic anticholinergic agent.

Central nervous system effects include delirium (disorientation to time and place accompanied by delusions, visual hallucinations and restlessness, anxiety and confusion) and possibly, seizures.

Peripheral effects will include rapid heart, dilatation of the pupils, decreased sweating, increased temperature (since the cooling mechanism of sweating is interfered with), decreased salivation, retention of urine, and decreased bowel activity. Of course, cardiac arrhythmias, as described above, may occur.

The patient will appear flushed, and his skin will feel warm and dry. His eyes will not tear. These physical signs help differentiate this toxic state from an acute psychotic break.

Such an overdose can be treated with the drug *physostigmine*. Physostigmine inhibits the action of cholinesterase, the enzyme which destroys acetylcholine. This permits a buildup of acetylcholine. Cholinergic transmission resumes, and the acute toxic symptoms subside. Physostigmine passes the blood-brain barrier so the central effects are relieved. Other drugs which may be used are the phenothiazines, to control confusion. and Valium and barbiturates, to control convulsions. Inderal may alleviate cardiac arrhythmias.

A syndrome similar to the one described above may also occur with overdoses of the antiparkinsonian agents, such as Cogentin and Artane. These drugs are also anticholinergic.

## THE MONOAMINE OXIDASE INHIBITORS (MAOI's)

This is the second major group of antidepressants. In most parts of the United States they are little used outside of hospitals. They have potentially serious side effects which have resulted in deaths.

Although these drugs are classified as inhibitors of a specific enzyme, monoamine oxidase, the clinician should be wary of ascribing their antidepressant effect only to that action. As is the case with most drugs, the MAOI's have many effects. They inhibit the enzymes which metabolize barbiturates, cocaine, alcohol, Demerol® (a powerful analgesic), and some anticholinergic drugs. Therefore, smaller doses of these drugs are employed if they are given simultaneously with the MAOI's.

### Mechanism of Action

As described above, the *tricyclics* act *outside* the neuron to prevent uptake of neurotransmitters. In contrast, the - *MAOI's* act *within* the neuron where they inhibit MAO (see Fig. 26). This enzyme is stored in submicroscopic structures called mitochondria. Apparently the MAOI's combine directly with MAO, preventing its deamination of the neurotransmitters serotonin, dopamine, epinephrine, and norepinephrine. The net effect is the increase of the concentrations of these transmitters in the brain.

## Types of MAOI's (see Table IV)

There are two main groups of MAOI's, based on their chemical structures. The first group to be discovered were derivatives of the chemical *hydrazine*. Hydrazine MAOI's were found to be toxic to the liver, so non-hydrazine types were sought. These types were found to be structurally related to amphetamine, the well-known stimulant and euphoriant (p. 146). For this reason, while the MAOI's have a long latency period before the antidepressant effect occurs, the non-hydrazine types are immediately stimulating and may cause excessive agitation, excitement, and inappropriate euphoria.

Table IV

Types of Monoamine Oxidase Inhibitors (MAOI'S)

| TYPE | DOSE |
|---|---|
| *Hydrazine MAOI's* | |
| Marplan (isocarboxazid) | 10 to 30 mg per day |
| Niamid® (nialamide) | 15 to 45 mg per day |
| | |
| *Nonhydrazine MAOI's* | |
| Eutonyl® (pargyline) | 25 to 200 mg per day |
| Parnate (tranylcypromine) | 10 to 30 mg per day |

The MAOI's are not considered as effective as the tricyclics in relieving depression. Some studies indicate they are little better than placebos. However, there may be certain types of depression for which they are indicated. They have been employed effectively in depressions in which the patient is severely retarded in his activity. They have also been used successfully in the treatment of phobic anxiety, and in patients with disabling obsessions. Some clinicians feel they have been underemployed; their popularity may increase.

## Absorption, Fate, and Excretion

MAOI's are rapidly absorbed when given orally. They pass to the liver, where much of their enzyme-inhibiting activity occurs, an undesirable feature. After metabolism, the metabolic products are excreted through the kidneys.

## Cardiovascular Effects

The MAOI's lower blood pressure, probably by blocking some excitatory nerve impulses to the heart. They have been used in cases of high blood pressure and angina pectoris, a condition related to coronary artery disease.

## CNS Effects

MAOI's increase the alerting action of the reticular formation, and increase the excitability of the amygdalae, midbrain structures which may mediate reward activity, as well as other functions.

## OTHER SIDE EFFECTS

The MAOI's have some anticholinergic type side effects, but the mechanism of action is not clear. A patient may experience difficulty in urination, inhibition of erection, impotence, and constipation. Allergic phenomenon may result in rashes and liver damage; the latter is rare.

More commonly, especially with the non-hydrazine MAOI's, the patient will experience excessive sympathetic stimulation, with dilatation of the pupils, agitation, increased temperature, and hallucinations and convulsions.

The most serious side effect of the MAOI's is elevation of blood pressure. This has caused hemorrhage of brain blood vessels with fifteen deaths, as of 1970.

If the MAOI's acted only in the brain, there would be no

problem. However, drugs do not go only to the sites where they produce their therapeutic effects. Unfortunately, the MAOI's inhibit MAO wherever they find it.

*Tyramine* is a substance which is found in many foods (see Food and Drug List below). In the normal person, it is absorbed from the G.I. tract and most of it is immediately metabolized by MAO, either in the liver or the intestinal wall. (MAO is found in many areas of the body.) However, if the patient is taking a MAOI, this fast metabolism does not occur, and the unchanged tyramine is free to circulate.

Foods and Drugs to Avoid When Taking MAOI's

Food: Cheeses — sharp and aged cheese; cream cheese and cottage cheese are acceptable.
Beer, wine — Chianti, sherry, others in large quantities
Pickled herring
Chicken livers
Yeast (bread o.k.)
Yogurt
Broad bean pods
Canned figs
Soy sauce
Snails
Sour cream
Chocolate
Creamed dishes
Avocado
Bananas
Cola drinks
Raisins

Drugs: Amphetamines
Caffeine
Ephedrine — a decongestant often found in nose drops and over-the-counter cold preparations
Methyldopa
Neo-Synephrine
Dopamine
Reserpine
Guanethedine

Tyramine acts to liberate norepinephrine from nerve endings. Norepinephrine, in turn, stimulates alpha-adrenergic receptors. This constricts blood vessels, increases the heart rate, and makes heart muscle contract more strongly. This, of course, results in an increase in blood pressure. In susceptible individuals, a weak blood vessel in the brain may rupture, causing a stroke.

This is the dangerous side effect which limits the usefulness of the MAOI's. Patients on them must eliminate the intake of foods which have a significant tyramine content (see p. 119).

Since many foods contain tyramine (cheese, cream dishes, wine, and beer), the patient is inconvenienced and may accidentally ingest tyramine. Often this will result in no worse than a headache, but a cerebral hemorrhage can occur, as described. A similar reaction may occur if the patient takes a drug which has a sympathomimetic effect. The drug's metabolism will be slowed by the MAOI. It will exert a hypertensive effect for an extended period, and with abnormally high intensity.

If a patient on an MAOI complains of headache, dizziness, rapid pulse or profuse sweating, his blood pressure should be taken immediately. If it is high (150/100 or above), the use of Regitine® (phentolamine), 5 mg I.V., should be considered. This drug blocks norepinephrine from reaching alpha-adrenergic sites, lowering the blood pressure.

## Combination With Tricyclics

Both the MAOI's and the tricyclics result in increased norepinephrine concentrations, and it was generally felt they should not be used in combination. In the past few years, cautious combinations in low dosages have been given successfully to depressed patients. The patient should be started on a tricyclic and the MAOI added cautiously, rather than starting with the MAOI and adding the tricyclic.

# CHAPTER 15

# LITHIUM

LITHIUM is unique. It is the first drug which can prevent an emotional illness before it happens. Unlike other psychiatric medications, lithium has no effect on mood, but stabilizes it within normal limits. To clarify this point, if a normal individual were to take lithium, he would be aware of no effect on his emotional state; if the same person were to take Thorazine, Elavil, or Valium, he would feel it.

Lithium is used in the treatment of manic-depressive psychosis. It is most successfully used to prevent episodes of mania. It is less consistently useful in the prevention of depression, but seems to be effective in some patients with recurring endogenous depression. It is also being tried in other emotional illnesses in which there are wide mood swings. It has been used successfully in patients with schizo-affective schizophrenia, a disease in which there is a mixture of schizophrenic and manic-depressive elements. It may be of value in other types of schizophrenia, when it is combined with standard antipsychotic drugs. It has also been tried, with varying degrees of success, in patients with alcoholism, heroin addiction, behavior disorders, tardive dyskinesia, and other psychiatric illnesses.

There are drawbacks to lithium. It does not work on all manic-depressives. It must be taken indefinitely, whether the patient is in a period of emotional illness or not. Regular blood levels must be done to determine if the lithium level is too high or too low. The therapeutic level is close to the toxic level. There may be long-term effects, such as thyroid disorder. The patient must be sincerely motivated to control his disease, cooperative, and alert for early signs of toxicity. These points will be discussed in more detail in this chapter.

Lithium is not a complex molecule. Rather, it is an element. It is in the same chemical family as sodium, potassium, rubidium, and cesium, the *alkali metals*. It was first discovered in 1817, and was used in the treatment of gout during the nineteenth century. Its antimanic properties were first discovered in 1949. It is usually administered as its carbonate salt, $Li_2CO_3$.

## Lithium Physiology

In the normal individual, there is no known biological role for lithium although trace amounts are present in the body. Lithium behaves like sodium in respect to its cellular action. A simplified account of some basic cell physiology is necessary to understand lithium action.

When a muscle cell is stimulated, sodium, which is present in the surrounding plasma, rushes in. Since sodium and lithium ions are positively charged, this changes the electrical potential between the inside and the outside of the cell. As sodium ions enter the cell, potassium ions leave it. This effect, *depolarization*, occurs during muscle contraction, and as an impulse travels along a peripheral nerve. The cell recovers from depolarization with the removal of the sodium by a mechanism known as the *sodium pump*, and the simultaneous inflow of potassium (see Fig. 27).

Lithium is not removed by the sodium-pump mechanism. If there is a low sodium concentration in the plasma or a high level of lithium, the cell may not repolarize normally. There would then be too much lithium intracellularly, and not enough potassium, which normally reenters as the sodium is pumped out. In the body muscles, this can lead to tremors and weakness. In cardiac muscle, it can lead to conduction deficits, arrhythmias,

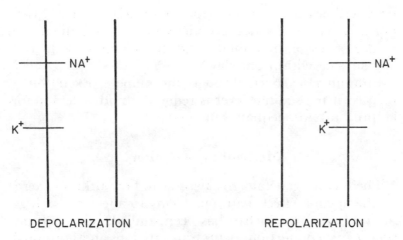

DEPOLARIZATION       REPOLARIZATION

Figure 27.

and other heart problems.

For this reason, the patient taking lithium must keep up an adequate salt and water intake. He generally should not be on diuretics, which eliminate salt and water from the body. Lithium must be used with extreme caution, if at all, with patients who have heart disease or significantly impaired kidney function. Every patient who may be placed on lithium should have a general physical exam, laboratory tests to determine if his serum levels of sodium and potassium are normal, kidney function tests, and, in older patients, an electrocardiogram (EKG).

## Absorption, Metabolism and Excretion

Lithium is readily absorbed from the intestinal tract. It is not bound to plasma proteins. It crosses the blood-brain barrier fairly easily, and its level in the brain is about 40 per cent of its level in the blood. It is absorbed completely within six to eight hours, and peak blood levels occur one to two hours after ingestion. Its half-life is about twenty-four hours. This means that one half of the lithium in the body will be excreted twenty-four hours after intake ceases. For this reason, if signs of toxicity occur, the patient can reduce or discontinue intake and the symptoms will usually subside within one day.

Lithium is excreted through the kidneys. Excretion is reduced if the sodium level is reduced, another reason for keeping up an adequate salt intake.

## Mechanism of Action

There is no general agreement as to how lithium exerts its therapeutic effect. Lithium seems to affect physiology in every area in which it has been studied; cellular function, nerve conduction, neurotransmission, and hormonal action. Perhaps its effect is dependent on more than one mechanism or is a result of some physiologic parameter as yet unstudied. (It should be reemphasized that this may apply to almost any psychotropic drug.)

At any rate, some effects of lithium are known. It decreases the sensitivity of dopamine receptors. It reduces brain catecholamine activity by increasing the reuptake of norepinephrine, dopamine and serotonin, thus acting opposite to the amphetamines and the tricyclic antidepressants. It inhibits the action of adenylcyclase, a cell membrane enzyme, which catalyzes the formation of a compound important in cellular metabolism. Adenylcyclase is important in serotonin synthesis and in dopamine receptors.

But, as outlined above, lithium also affects peripheral nerve and muscle cells, changing their conduction properties, excitability, and the cellular concentrations of sodium and potassium. Since lithium may substitute for sodium and potassium, it may affect a host of enzymatic actions which are sodium and potassium dependent.

Lithium also affects hormonal activity, as shown by its long-term effect on the thyroid gland (see Table V).

Table V

Toxic Effects of Lithium

| Serum Level | Toxic Effects |
|---|---|
| 1.6 - 3.0 | Tremor, nausea,* diarrhea,* abdominal pain, excessive thirst,* increased urination,* vomiting, ringing in ears, blurred vision, drowsiness, stumbling gait, EKG changes |
| 2.0 - 4.0 | Muscle spasms and weakness, jerky eye movements, confusion, slurred speech, pulse irregularities, fall in blood pressure, convulsions |
| 4.0 and above | Death from irreversible kidney damage or pulmonary infection as a result of coma |

Possible long-term effects not related to serum level:

Enlargement of thyroid gland with or without decreased thyroid functioning: loss of ability to concentrate urine resulting in greatly increased thirst and voluminous urination (diabetes insipidus); increased white cell count; cogwheel rigidity of arms (extrapyramidal symptoms); birth defects such as malformation of the heart; acnelike skin eruption.

At least one investigator feels that the long term use of lithium may induce a loss of ambition, lack of engagement in work, and general listlessness. This, at present, is only a preliminary clinical impression and needs further study.

*may also occur at lower levels

## Clinical Use of Lithium

Lithium is usually administered in 300 mg capsules. The dosage may range from 600 mg per day to 2400 mg per day.

When treating a patient in acute mania, six to ten days are necessary for full effect. A phenothiazine, such as

Thorazine, is usually administered simultaneously. There is no reason why the two drugs cannot be used together.

A curious, but clinically important, fact is that an acutely manic patient can tolerate a higher dose of lithium than he can after the mania is broken. This is important because toxicity can develop rapidly if dosage is not reduced after the mania is controlled. An acutely manic patient may absorb 1800 mg of lithium a day without ill effect, and show a blood level less than 1.5 meq/l. When the mania breaks, the same dosage may produce a much higher level. The ability of the acutely manic patient to absorb large amounts of lithium has not been explained, but should be kept in mind. There have been cases of patients going into coma on doses of lithium which they had tolerated well when acutely manic.

After control of mania is achieved, the dosage is readjusted to maintain a level between .8 and 1.2. There are patients who get excellent therapeutic effect on much lower blood levels, as well as those who get toxic at lower levels, but most patients require a level of at least .8 for therapeutic effect. During the initial phase of lithium treatment, frequent blood levels are taken. After a maintenance dose is established, monthly levels are usually sufficient. Of course, if signs of toxicity, mania, or depression occur, a level should be taken immediately. A yearly thyroid test and an occasional serum sodium and potassium are in order.

Lithium can be started between attacks of mania or depression. Usually a "loading dose" of 600 mg three times a day is given, followed by a maintenance dose between 600 and 900 mg per day. Elderly patients usually excrete lithium more slowly, and their dosages are correspondingly reduced.

### Side Effects (Table V)

Lithium is not anticholinergic. It is not sedative or

stimulating. However, it can have serious side effects and, as mentioned above, the therapeutic level is close to the toxic level. In this respect, it differs from other psychotropic medications which usually have a wide range of dosage safety.

The patient can learn to monitor side effects, reducing or discontinuing his dosage if they appear. He should be taught to recognize early signs of toxicity. Nausea often occurs during the first few days of treatment and can be relieved by taking the medication with food. If it occurs later in treatment, it may then be a sign of toxicity. Vomiting, diarrhea, and tremor must all be watched for (see Table V). The patient should be warned to keep up salt and water intake. He should not go on diuretics while on lithium. Lithium toxicity is more likely to occur during a bout of acute infectious illness. Fever, diarrhea, and vomiting can lead to dehydration and salt imbalance, precipitating lithium toxicity.

The mechanisms of most lithium side effects are not fully known. It may be speculated, however, that excessive lithium interferes with normal peripheral and central neuronal conduction, causing tremor, ataxia, confusion, slurred speech, and coma. The interference with normal muscle cell excitability can account for muscle weakness and fatigue. Disruptions in normal potassium level may have serious effects on heart action, probably accounting for electrocardiogram (EKG) changes, arrhythmias, and hypotension.

Routine blood levels should be taken about twelve hours after the last lithium dosage. The patient should be instructed not to take a morning dose on the day he is to have a blood level.

# CHAPTER 16

# THE MINOR TRANQUILIZERS

MINOR TRANQUILIZER is a term which has become entrenched in psychopharmacology. It is defined as a psychotropic medication which may be indicated in nonpsychotic conditions such as neuroses, situational crises, and personality disorders. (The drugs used for psychoses are *major tranquilizers,* although many of them do not tranquilize; their important action is antipsychotic.) The term *tranquilizer* was coined to distinguish a newer class of compounds from the older sedatives, such as the barbiturates (see Chapter 17). Drugs classified as sedatives induce sleep or slow activity. Tranquilizing drugs are said to reduce anxiety, without reducing arousal state. Thus, they may relieve anxiety without reducing overall performance or causing sleep.

## THE BENZODIAZEPINES

The most widely used group of minor tranquilizers, the *benzodiazepines,* share several characteristics which make them useful in a variety of conditions: (1) relaxation of voluntary muscles; (2) taming of aggressive behavior; (3) anticonvulsant action; and (4) reduction of anxiety.

Anxiety is a state in which there is a feeling of impending doom. All is not right with the world; what is wrong cannot be clearly defined. Anxiety may be transient and easily repressed, or so overwhelming as to immobilize the person. It is part of the clinician's job to distinguish normal anxiety, which may be a healthy response to the world and the self, from abnormally painful apprehension deserving drug treatment.

The benzodiazepines have other medical uses. They are important in the treatment of alcohol withdrawal, exerting an anticonvulsant, as well as calming, effect. Some chronic alcoholics are able to maintain sobriety by substituting Valium for alcohol. They are also useful in cardiac patients because of the low incidence of cardiac side effects. They have been used successfully in behavior disorders characterized by explosive, uncontrolled violence.

## General Effects of the Benzodiazepines

The commonly prescribed benzodiazepines are Valium (diazepam), Librium (chlordiazepoxide), Serax (oxazepam), Tranxene (clorazepate), and Dalmane® (flurazepam). They will be discussed as a group. While there are differences between them, the differences are minor. However, some patients will report feeling better on one than on another, especially Valium, which outsells all the others.

As mentioned above, the benzodiazepines reduce anxiety without decreasing arousal. Their main action is in the brain itself. They act to reduce neuronal activity in the midbrain, depressing the septal structures, the amygdalae, and the hippocampus (see p. 46). They inhibit hypothalamic nuclei and thalamic structures and suppress the ascending reticular activating system. In the spinal cord, they inhibit spinal reflexes, probably an important component of their muscle-relaxant effect.

The molecular mechanism by which benzodiazapines act is not clear. One animal study indicates they may mimic glycine, a neurotransmitter in the spinal cord, brain stem, and thalamus. Librium may interfere with the conversion of DOPA to dopamine in the neuron and may counteract the effect of dopamine outside the neuron. Some work indicates that the benzodiazepines block activity in limbic structures in which serotonin is a neuro-transmitter.

As discussed in the section on the limbic system (see p. 45), there are structures in this area which mediate the behavior and the feelings associated with punishment and reward, withdrawal and aggression. The benzodiazepines may block impulses in the structures which mediate angry and aggressive behavior or reactions associated with fear.

The concept of neurotransmitters systems acting in balance may be crucial. The benzodiazepines may help restore an imbalance between systems having to do with aggression and withdrawal. At any rate, the presence of a benzodiazepine or its active metabolites in the midbrain reduces the feeling of anxiety which may color the patient's activities. It also reduces behavior associated with rage.

### Absorption, Fate, and Excretion

The benzodiazepines are well absorbed from the gut and may also be administered by the intramuscular or intravenous route. Surprisingly, intramuscularly injected Valium and Librium do not reach as high blood concentrations as they do when taken orally, nor are they as rapidly absorbed. They are bound to plasma proteins. There are high plasma levels one to two hours after oral administration, but clinical effects may be felt within a half hour. The half-life is about twenty-four hours, so the duration of action is fairly long. An exception to this is Serax, which has a short half-life of three to twenty hours. Some clinicians feel that, as with the phenothiazines, the benzodiazepines, except for Serax, may be given at bedtime and the antianxiety effect will persist through the following day.

Metabolites may be detected in the urine two weeks after administration has ceased. Valium has an enterohepatic circulation which probably prolongs its action.

The benzodiazepines are metabolized by demethylation, hydroxylation, and conjugation in the liver. The metabolites themselves may be quite active. For example, Tranxene is metabolized mainly to nordiazepam, the compound which probably exerts its desired clinical effect. Serax is the metabolite into which Valium and Librium are transformed. The benzodiazepines are excreted mainly by the kidneys but about one-fifth is excreted in the feces.

## Preparations

Benzodiazepines are usually administered as capsules, but intramuscular and intravenous injectable forms are available. The latter are valuable when the patient is unable to take oral medications.

## Side Effects (see Table VI)

The benzodiazepines are generally safe drugs. It is almost impossible to take a fatal overdose of any of them unless there is simultaneous ingestion of alcohol, barbiturates, or some other drug which depresses respiration. Then the presence of the benzodiazepine may increase the effect of the other drug to the point of a fatal result.

However, a large number of undesirable side effects have been reported with these drugs. They are summarized in Table VI. There is little understanding of the mechanisms of these side effects. For example, although the benzodiazepines are known not to be anticholinergic, dry mouth and constipation has been observed with them. This may be due to their stimulation of sympathetic activity, which would slow down the gut and cause secretion of thickened saliva (see Table I).

Both urinary retention and loss of urinary control have been attributed to the benzodiazepines. They also produce various allergic symptoms, presumably by antigenic stim-

Table VI

Side Effects of the Benzodiazepines

| | |
|---|---|
| Neurological | Addiction, increased appetite, respiratory arrest (very rare), ataxia, confusion, depression, euphoria, excitement, extra-pyramidal symptoms (very rare), fatigue, fever, hallucinations, headache, insomnia, irritability, increased or decreased libido, nightmares, seizures during withdrawal, physical and psychological dependence |
| Allergic | Agranulocytosis, conjunctivitis, jaundice, liver damage, leukopenia, neutropenia |
| Heart and Vessels | Edema, hypotension, syncope (fainting), tachycardia (rapid heart), thrombophlebitis |
| Endocrine | Failure to ovulate, menstrual irregularities, weight gain |
| Gastrointestinal | Constipation, dry mouth, nausea |
| Genito-urinary | Loss of bladder control, retention of urine, abnormal kidney tests |
| Ocular | Blurred vision, diplopia (double vision) |
| Miscellaneous | Suicidal depression in patients taking over 40 mg per day of Valium (rare), increased effects of MAO inhibitors, tricyclics, phenothiazines, barbiturates and narcotics, intoxication of newborn infants who may display respiratory abnormalities, lethargy, and poor muscle tone |

ulation, as discussed in Chapter 11. An unusual allergic reaction to Valium is *conjunctivitis,* or burning and redness of the membranes of the eye.

The neurological side effects are the most common. In fairly low doses they may produce *ataxia,* a stumbling gait, uncertainty of arm and hand movements, and slurred speech. This is probably due to their depressant effect on subcortical structures such as the cerebellum. Unlike the barbiturates, they are not thought to depress the cortex. Drowsiness is also a fairly common side effect.

There has also been a report of a state of organic psychosis with visual hallucinations, restlessness, mania, confusion, euphoria, and memory deficit in an elderly patient who took only 30 mg of Dalmane. The mechanism is unclear; presumably, benzodiazepines affect normal neurotransmitter activity.

The benzodiazepines may be habit-forming to the point of addiction. Because of the twenty to twenty-four hour half-life, tissue levels rise as the drug is taken day after day (see p. 75). Tolerance to these drugs develops. That is, with prolonged administration the same dosage will produce less effect. There is progressive diminution of effect with continued administration, so more of the drug must be taken to produce the euphoric tranquility some patients may seek. An addiction-prone individual, usually one with very low tolerance for anxiety, may therefore take excessive amounts of Valium for a long period.

When the individual tries to go off the drug, a syndrome of intense anxiety and restlessness may ensue. There have been rare cases of convulsions in patients stopping very high doses. The drug may dampen normal brain activity to the point that, when it is no longer present, even minor stimuli may trigger seizure. The brain's neurons become highly sensitive due to having been "screened" for so long by the drug.

To reduce the chance of psychological or physiological dependence, the benzodiazepines should be taken on a p.r.n. basis, and not on an automatic daily schedule. The patient should learn to take them only when his anxiety is intolerable or when it seriously impairs his performance. He should strive to lower his dose, not maintain it. This is in contrast to the antidepressants and antipsychotics, which must be taken regularly over a long period in adequate dosage.

The non-medical practitioner will rarely deal with a patient who requires intravenous Valium. However, it is well to mention that there have been occasional cases of thrombophlebitis with I.V. Valium. This means that a clot forms in the vein at the site of the injection. As it usually occurs several days after injection, the non-medical clinician may see it. This complication may occur because Valium is not very soluble in water, so some solid material may inadvertently enter the vein, forming a core point for a clot to develop. Any patient complaining of pain, swelling or redness at the point of a recent injection of Valium (or any drug), should be checked for thrombophlebitis.

## THE HYDROXYZINES

There are only two main tranquilizers in this chemical group. Their trade names are Atarax and Vistaril. They are little used, in comparison with the benzodiazepines. However, they are non-habit-forming, are good sedatives, and have a place in mental health practice.

The hydroxyzines are antihistaminic (see p. 63). Many antihistamines have sedative effects. The sedative effect is not necessarily due to the antihistaminic effect. The precise mechanism of action of the hydroxyzines is unknown; the histamine-blocking action may not be important.

In addition to being antihistaminic, this group is weakly anticholinergic. Tranquilizing action may be due to a central anticholinergic effect. Hydroxyzines suppress activity in the ascending reticular activating system of the brain stem and the hypothalamus. As is the case with the benzodiazepines, their action is subcortical. Thus, in low doses, they reduce anxiety without reducing mental alertness or wakefulness. At higher doses, they may be effective sleep medications.

The hydroxyzines are useful in relieving anxiety associated with some physical illnesses, such as skin conditions and intestinal tract disorders. They have been used beneficially in behavior disorders and alcoholism, and are particularly useful in patients who have an addictive potential. Unlike the benzodiazepines, whose sedative effects have been compared to alcohol, they do not induce euphoria, and therefore, are not especially pleasant to take.

Side effects also reduce their addictive potential. They are mildly anticholinergic and so may cause dry mouth and blurred vision. Some patients complain of a feeling of mental "fuzziness" and/or inner restlessness, possibly pointing to some extrapyramidal effects. There have been cases of convulsions in patients taking large amounts. Hydroxyzines probably lower the convulsive threshold, in contrast to the benzodiazepines which are anticonvulsant.

Unlike almost all other psychotropic drugs, no serious side effects in the liver or blood have been reported from hydroxyzines' usage. There have been rare cases of allergic skin conditions, however. Again unlike the benzodiazepines, tolerance does not develop with Atarax or Vistaril. They may be taken in the same doses indefinitely, usually 25 to 300 mg a day, with no loss of antianxiety effect.

The hydroxyzines are well absorbed from the intestinal tract, and may be administered intramuscularly but not intravenously. Their metabolic fate and half-life are not established.

On the whole, the hydroxyzines may be the safest minor tranquilizers now available for long-term use.

### MEPROBAMATE

Meprobamate was the first drug to which the name tranquilizer was applied. It was marketed in 1954, and eagerly sought by the public and prescribed by physicians, who were glad to have a nonbarbiturate drug for anxiety. By many measurements, meprobamate (Miltown, Equanil) is no better than the barbiturates; it shares many of their advantages and disadvantages.

Meprobamate is a member of the chemical group *dicarbamates*. There are other members of this group used as tranquilizers and muscle relaxants: Tybatran®, Colacen® (tybamate); Soma® and Rela® (carisopradol). However, meprobamate is the most widely used, so the discussion of the dicarbamates will be limited to meprobamate.

## General Effects

The effects of meprobamate depend on the dosage given. At low-dosage, 200 to 400 mg, sedation occurs. *Sedation* may be defined as the decreased response of an organism to a constant level of stimulation. This is the desired effect, as it is usually accompanied by a decrease in subjective feelings of anxiety.

At therapeutic doses, 400 to 1600 mg/day, there is no apparent effect on cortical structures. The drug acts in the midbrain, hypothalamus, thalamus, and basal ganglia. Its molecular action is unknown. There is no known effect on cholinergic or adrenergic neurotransmission.

However, at higher doses there is apparently some cortical depression, which is manifested by euphoria, impaired judgment, and loss of self-control. In this respect, meprobamate may be compared to alcohol and barbiturates. Like them, it is potentially addicting, tolerance can develop, and serious withdrawal states may occur.

## Preparations

Meprobamate is usually given by tablet, occasionally by liquid concentrate. There is no injectable form.

## Absorption, Fate, and Excretion

The drug is well absorbed from the intestinal tract, reaching peak levels in one to two hours. It is metabolized in the liver by hydroxylation. An interesting and possibly clinically important phenomena is that meprobamate stimulates the enzymes which metabolize it, thus hastening its own metabolism. This may partially explain meprobamate tolerance: A patient may gradually build up to enormous dosages without experiencing sedation.

The half-life of meprobamate is about ten hours. Drugs with half-lives in the ten to twenty-four hour range often are characterized by severe withdrawal syndromes. This is because while the drug is being ingested high tissue levels can build up. When ingestion ceases, the tissue level falls fairly quickly. Drugs with half-lives of six to eight hours seldom accumulate to high tissue levels. Drugs with a thirty-six to forty-eight hour half-life may accumulate to high tissue levels, but the level will fall slowly when ingestion ceases, allowing time for the body to adjust. These points are also important with the barbiturates, as will be discussed (p. 142).

Meprobamate is excreted mainly in the urine.

## Side Effects

The most commonly reported side effect is drowsiness. Other CNS effects, presumably due to depression of normal neural activity, include ataxia, dizziness, paradoxical excitement, weakness, and paralysis of eye muscles.

The most serious common adverse reaction is the withdrawal syndrome. This occurs when a patient who has been taking excessive amounts for long periods, thus building up a tolerance, suddenly stops intake. This may occur when he runs out of the drug and can get no more, is hospitalized, or has a psychotic episode. Patients have been reported taking up to eighty 400 mg tablets a day.

The severity of the withdrawal syndrome depends on the amount habitually taken. With patients taking relatively small doses, the syndrome may be characterized by disturbed sleep, with excess dreaming. Progressively severe withdrawals are characterized by restlessness, weakness, tremor, increased blood pressure, rapid pulse and respiration, and convulsions. Toxic psychoses with agitation, confusion, and hallucinations may occur.

Rare allergic reactions have been reported to meprobamate, and there may be cross allergies with other members of the dicarbamate family. The mechanisms are probably the same as those described elsewhere (Chapter 11). A patient may develop urticaria or other skin eruptions. If the allergic response centers in the blood system, serious blood dyscrasias may occur: aplastic anemia, thrombocytopenia, leukopenia, agranulocytosis, and red cell depression. A toxic syndrome with edema and fever has been seen, possibly due to the histamine release associated with allergic reactions. These reactions usually occur early in treatment.

Gastrointestinal side effects to meprobamate include nausea, vomiting, and diarrhea. The mechanism of these effects is not clear.

The cardiovascular system may also be affected. EKG changes have been observed. Some patients have developed irregular heart rhythms and severe lowering of blood pressure, resulting in at least one fatality.

Although the above recital of side effects has a frightening sound, the serious reactions are rare and generally treatable by withdrawal of the drug and institution of appropriate medical treatment. The non-medical practitioner should be aware that meprobamate is an abusable drug and that serious side effects are possible. A final cautionary note is that it may tend to deepen depression in an already depressed patient.

## Uses of Meprobamate

Taken briefly, and only as needed, it is a useful antianxiety drug. It is also of value as a sleep medication, but again, only temporarily. Rarely, it has been of some value in psychotic patients, but it does not ameliorate delusions or hallucinations.

# CHAPTER 17

# THE BARBITURATES

THIS group of drugs is little used in modern psychiatry. The barbiturates have been almost completely replaced as antianxiety drugs by the minor tranquilizers. Some older patients, especially those with concomitant medical problems, continue to take them. Unfortunately, the barbiturates are commonly taken illicitly; a discussion of them would almost be more appropriate in a text on drug abuse.

The barbiturates (see Table VII) have been in clinical use for over seventy years, and is a complex and well-studied group of drugs. Their metabolism is intricate, some aspects beyond the appropriate scope of the non-medical practitioner. For this reason, the following account will be somewhat oversimplified and, in comparison with the amount known about barbiturates, incomplete.

## General Effects

The antianxiety drugs discussed in the previous chapter generally affect midbrain and related subcortical structures. Only in high doses do they measurably affect the cortex or brain stem. Barbiturates are different. They affect almost all of the CNS, *beginning* with the cortex and the reticular activating system. They tend to depress neural activity. The mechanism of this, at the submicroscopic level, is to decrease the excitability of the pre- and postsynaptic membranes. They may also interfere with neurotransmission.

When a barbiturate is given, there is an initial increase

Table VII

Barbiturates

Long-Acting

| *Trade Name* | *Chemical Name* |
|---|---|
| Luminal,® Probital® | Phenobarbital |
| Mebaral® | Mephabarbital |

Intermediate and Short-Acting

| | |
|---|---|
| Amytal® | Amobarbital |
| Butisol® | Butabarbital |
| Nembutal | Pentobarbital |
| Seconal | Secobarbital |
| Tuinal | Secobarbital-Amobarbital |

NOTE: There are many drugs which contain one or more barbiturates as one of their ingredients. This table lists only a few pure barbiturate drugs.

of cortical activity because of a decrease in the inhibiting effect of the reticular activating system. This is followed by depression of the stimulating effects of the reticular input, along with a general depression of cortical activity. Thus, they induce an imbalance between inhibiting and activating systems in the brain. A patient may therefore experience a transitory euphoria, which is followed by a dulling of his sensorium.

Since the barbiturates act at all levels of the brain, they cannot be considered antianxiety drugs in the same sense that drugs which act mainly in the limbic areas are. Some patients experience excitement, and others, depression, on barbiturates. The euphoria and excitement, as well as the sedative effects, may account for the wide spectrum of abuse. The barbiturates are like alcohol: They deinhibit, cause transient euphoria, and dull unpleasant emotions. Like alcohol, they are addicting; severe withdrawal symptoms may occur and, if taken in sufficient quantity, death may result from respiratory depression.

## Preparations

The barbiturates have legitimate medical uses other than in psychiatry. They have a respectable place as anticonvulsants, are of great value in anesthesia, and may be of brief, appropriate use in cases of insomnia. Over the years, they have been marketed as powders, elixirs, syrups, drops, suppositories, capsules, tablets, in sustained and delayed release forms, and as injectables. They also have the virtue of being inexpensive.

## Absorption, Fate, and Excretion

Barbiturates are classified according to their length of action. The long-acting forms have half-lives of twenty-four to ninety-six hours, but are clinically effective for only six to twelve hours. The short- to intermediate-acting forms have fourteen to forty-two hour half-lives, and are clinically effective for about six to eight hours. There are ultrashort-acting forms, used almost exclusively in anesthesia, which have a half-life of three to eight hours but whose clinical effect may be as short as fifteen minutes.

It is the short and intermediate acting forms which are usually employed as antianxiety or sleep medications. The long-acting forms are mainly used as anticonvulsants (Table VII).

The barbiturates may be given orally, rectally, or by

injection. They are bound to plasma proteins. They are distributed to all body tissues: They appear in the milk of nursing mothers. One of the factors affecting their distribution is the extent to which they dissolve in lipids (fats). Cell membranes contain lipids, and there is a high concentration of lipids in the brain. The more highly lipid-soluble barbiturates are shorter acting and have a rapid onset of action. They bind to tissue proteins as well as plasma proteins. Very short acting compounds are short acting because the drug at first concentrates in the brain, then leaves the brain as it is taken up by muscle and fat. There is a slow release of the barbiturate by muscle and fat after the acute effect has passed. This phenomenon probably accounts for barbiturate "hangover."

The barbiturates are metabolized by various enzymatic reactions in the liver. They are powerful inducers of liver enzymes: they stimulate the action of the enzymes which metabolize them. They also stimulate enzymes which metabolize other drugs, a recently appreciated action which may lead to clinical complications.

For example, a patient may be put on Coumadin®, a medication which lengthens the clotting time of blood. If he is simultaneously taking a barbiturate, it will induce enzymes which metabolize Coumadin. Higher doses of Coumadin will be necessary to achieve the desired lengthening of clotting time. If the patient then stops taking the barbiturate, the dose of Coumadin will be too high. If it is not reduced, serious bleeding problems may arise.

The phenomenon of tolerance to barbiturates is due to two main factors. Barbiturates induce enzymes for their own metabolism, and nervous tissue becomes resistant to their effects. The latter tolerance factor probably comes about by an increase in the number and/or sensitivity of central nervous system receptors which the drug blocks. This phenomenon, *pharmacodynamic tolerance*, probably occurs with many other drugs.

Most barbiturates depend on liver metabolism for termination of their action. The main exception is phenobarbital, thirty per cent of which is excreted unchanged in the urine. Thus, in patients with liver disease who need a barbiturate, phenobarbital is the drug of choice, but it should be avoided in patients with impaired kidney function.

## Side Effects

The usual spectrum of psychotropic side effects occurs with barbiturates: drowsiness, ataxia, paradoxical excitement, and allergic reactions. However, no autonomic side effects are characteristic.

Of serious concern is the respiratory depression which may occur with overdose. It is beyond the scope of the non-medical practitioner to advise or treat overdosage of barbiturates. This almost always requires hospital treatment in an intensive care unit.

Death is more likely to result from barbiturate overdosage than from any other psychotropic medication. The mechanism of death is usually related to the barbiturates' ability to depress neural activity at all levels of the brain. Since maintenance of respiration is dependent on several neural mechanisms, a high-enough concentration of barbiturates may depress these areas to the point of respiratory paralysis. Even before this point is reached, respiration may be so depressed that oxygenation of tissues is inadequate, with resultant damage to brain, heart and other tissues.

Severe withdrawal reactions may occur in patients who are taking high quantities of the intermediate-acting barbiturates, such as Tuinal®, Nembutal®, and Seconal®. Depending on the habitual amount, withdrawal syndromes may range from jitteriness and ataxia to psychotic excitement, delirium and grand mal epileptic convulsions.

While extremely alarming to the patient and witnesses, a convulsion by itself is not necessarily harmful. Harm may come if the vicitm bites his tongue or if he vomits and sucks the vomitus into the lungs, causing pneumonia or strangulation. He may injure himself falling or thrashing, or lie unconscious unattended in a dangerous position.

The actual convulsion itself — the period of excessive CNS discharge spreading from a sensitive focus — is not in itself dangerous. As long as the patient's respiration is maintained and he does not injure himself, after the convulsion he will sleep, and awaken as usual.

Occasionally, a state of continuous convulsion may occur, *status epilepticus*, but this usually happens in cases of chronic epilepsy, not drug withdrawal. In status epilepticus, there is danger of brain damage from prolonged insufficient oxygenation.

# CHAPTER 18

# STIMULANTS

$S$TIMULANT drugs have had a generally bad press for some years. Once hailed as an effective treatment for fatigue, obesity, and depression, the amphetamines are now almost outlaw drugs. Their potential for abuse is well known and use in psychiatry is minimal.

There are some clinicians who feel that the rejection of the stimulant drugs may have gone too far. Certainly, they are useful in the hyperkinetic syndrome of childhood (minimal brain dysfunction or MBD), even though their effect is, paradoxically, to sedate rather than arouse. Judicious use of amphetamine has been of some value for geriatric patients who display apathy, low energy, and excessive sleep. There is also a neurological entity, narcolepsy, in which the patient may sleep almost continuously because of a CNS lesion. Amphetamines are the treatment of choice for narcolepsy.

This section will briefly describe four stimulant drugs: Amphetamine, Ritalin (methylphenidate), Cylert® (pemoline), and caffeine. Their pharmacology provides a useful review of the sympathetic nervous system. Stimulant drugs generally stimulate sympathetic nervous activity either by direct action on adrenergic receptors, or stimulation of sympathetic nerves. They also increase adrenergic activity in the brain.

## AMPHETAMINES

### General Effects

Amphetamines have been employed since 1935 in the

146

treatment of narcolepsy, a neurological disorder characterized by frequent, irresistible, daytime sleep. They were also used and misused as a stimulant to ward off fatigue, and to increase alertness. Their appetite-suppressant effect is utilized in the treatment of obesity. They have been used as antidepressants because of their stimulant and euphoriant qualities, but are not considered a true antidepressant, since they are stimulants rather than mood normalizers. Of course, amphetamines are potentially addicting, and the patient may suffer increased depression after they are withdrawn.

Amphetamine apparently acts mainly in the brain stem reticular formation and the hypothalamus. It increases activity in the ascending reticular formation and in the midbrain. This indirectly increases cortical activity but it may also have a direct effect on the cortex too. In the peripheral nervous system amphetamine has a *sympathomimetic* effect (see Table I): The pupils dilate, blood vessels constrict, heart rate increases, there is increased release of sugar from the liver, the sphincter of the bladder tightens, and the bronchial muscles relax. The effect on the intestinal tract is unpredictable. Both constipation and diarrhea may occur.

Amphetamines act in several ways at the molecular level. They release dopamine and norepinephrine from presynaptic neurons, and inhibit reuptake of the released catecholamines. They also inhibit MAO, and may have a direct effect as neurotransmitters, stimulating postsynaptic receptors.

## Preparations

Amphetamines are marketed as a tablet, a long-acting spansule, and an elixir. Various other preparations, such as methamphetamine, "speed" can be given by injection.

## Absorption, Fate and Excretion

Amphetamines are rapidly absorbed from the G.I. tract and easily cross the blood-brain barrier. They are metabolized mainly in the liver, and the metabolic products are eliminated in the urine.

## Side Effects

Many side effects of amphetamine are really extremes of its normal actions; restlessness, irritability, tension, insomnia, weight loss, confusion, increased libido, convulsions, and other signs of excess stimulation of the CNS. In the G.I. tract, dry mouth, vomiting, diarrhea, and cramps may occur. The cardiovascular system may display heart irregularities, angina, excess sweating, and high blood pressure, which may lead to cerebral hemorrhage. A rare, but very serious, complication has been described in patients on therapeutic doses, as well as in abusers. It consists of degeneration of arterial vessels, with resultant organ and tissue damage; a *necrotizing vasculitis*.

Severe amphetamine intoxication may lead to *amphetamine psychosis*, which closely mimics, and may be indistinguishable from, acute schizophrenia. There are paranoid auditory and visual hallucinations, excitement, and repetitive stereotyped behavior. It has been theorized that dopamine excess is largely responsible for this chemical psychosis. As is true in schizophrenia, this syndrome may be treated by the dopamine-blocking major tranquilizers.

Allergy to the amphetamines may occur and reactions such as urticaria have been observed.

## Uses

As mentioned above, generally accepted use of the

amphetamines is now limited. In minimal brain dysfunction amphetamines have been largely replaced by Ritalin. Dextroamphetamine is the treatment of choice for narcolepsy, but this is a neurological, rather than a psychiatric, condition. However, low doses of amphetamine (5 to 10 mg two or three times a day) may be useful in withdrawn, listless patients. Thus, it may be useful in some geriatric patients. Another use to which amphetamine may be put is in the treatment of enuresis. It acts to lighten sleep and also to contract the sphincter of the urinary bladder.

### RITALIN (Methylphenidate)

Ritalin has become the drug of choice for the hyperkinetic syndrome of childhood or MBD. This disease is characterized by short attention span, hyperactivity with purposeless, restless movement, emotional lability, poor self-control, clumsy gait, and difficulty with fine motor movements. There may be other soft neurological signs. In children who are accurately diagnosed as having MBD, Ritalin will produce remarkable improvement. The child becomes tractable, calm, and less moody. His intellectual and peer performance improves. His emotional state tends to reflect reality rather than inner turmoil.

How does a stimulant drug exert this apparently paradoxical effect? Current theory holds that MBD children may have damage to ascending tracts in the reticular activating system (RAS), possibly caused by inadequate oxygenation at birth. The damaged tracts normally carry input to the brain from the external environment. If they malfunction, the child may be overwhelmed either by a flood of irrelevant data or, possibly, understimulated by a lack of relevant data.

In any case, Ritalin probably normalizes function in the reticular activating system. Tracts which carry incoming data are affected, as well as tracts which have an inhibitory effect on cortical function. Thus, the stimulant drug is essentially stimulating *underaroused* areas of the RAS. The behavioral effect is a reduction of restless, purposeless activity. Usually, Ritalin treatment may be discontinued in adolescence, and often much earlier. This may be due to physiological maturation of the central nervous system, which compensates for earlier deficits.

The molecular action of Ritalin is to release dopamine and norepinephrine in the CNS. It also blocks uptake of the monoamines. In these actions, it is similar to amphetamine. However, it has far less peripheral effect than amphetamine and less stimulation of motor activity. Its molecular structure is similar to the amphetamines, and it shares a potential for abuse; Ritalin induces euphoria and increased energy.

## Preparations and Dosage

Ritalin is marketed as a tablet. It has been used in injectable form in experimental work. The usual dose is 10 to 60 mg per day, given after meals, in order to minimize its effect as an appetite suppressant.

## Absorption, Fate, and Excretion

The absorption, metabolism, and excretion of Ritalin is similar to amphetamine (see p. 148). A single dose is completely eliminated as the parent drug, or its metabolites, in twenty-four hours.

## Side Effects

In children, use of Ritalin has been associated with decreased rate of growth and decreased rate of weight gain. This is probably related to its effect on the appetite controls of the hypothalamus, reducing food craving. It may also be due to direct interference with growth hormone (see p. 52).

If Ritalin is given to a schizophrenic patient, he may respond with increased psychotic process, hostility and rage. Ritalin increases activation and decreases inhibition in manic patients. These effects, incidentally, may be reversed by giving physostigmine, a drug which increases brain acetylcholine (see p. 115). Since the effect of Ritalin (and other sympathomimetics) is to increase dopamine and norepinephrine transmission, this again points to the balance of neurotransmitter systems in the brain. Giving physostigmine presumably increases acetylcholine transmission which would tend to balance excessive dopaminergic transmission.

Ritalin also inhibits the metabolism of certain drugs, such as Dilantin, phenobarbital, and the tricyclic antidepressants. These drugs must be given in reduced dosages when Ritalin is administered.

As with the amphetamines, a spectrum of unwanted effects may occur which are extremes of its therapeutic action: Loss of appetite (anorexia), restlessness, insomnia, hyperactivity, excitement and convulsions may occur. A susceptible patient may become psychotic. An overdose may cause a toxic psychosis.

Allergic reactions may also occur, including skin eruptions and blood dyscrasias.

Cardiac abnormalities, such as high blood pressure and arrhythmias, have been observed.

## Other Uses

In addition to MDB, Ritalin is of value in narcolepsy. It may also be useful in treating the apathy and withdrawal seen in some geriatric patients or senile individuals.

## CYLERT (Pemoline)

This new drug is just coming on the market for use in MBD. Cylert is structurally different from amphetamine and Ritalin.

Its manufacturer claims it can be given in once-a-day dosage, and that cardiovascular and neurological side effects are insignificant. Initial weight loss has occurred in children on the drug, but has returned to normal within a few months.

The drug apparently acts to increase release of dopamine, possibly by stimulating its synthesis.

Its serum half-life is twelve hours. It is excreted by the kidneys, 75 per cent of an oral dose appearing in the urine in twenty-four hours. Side effects observed so far include psychotic reactions in abusers, allergic reactions damaging the liver, skin rash, anorexia, dizziness, headache, stomach ache, and hallucinations.

## CAFFEINE

Caffeine may be useful in certain disorders, such as MBD. It is a ubiquitous drug, to which most Americans and Europeans are addicted. The average cup of coffee contains 100 to 150 mg of caffeine, and comparable amounts are present in tea and cola drinks. To go through the pharmacology of this very common drug may add to the sophistication of the non-medical practitioner. It may serve to emphasize that psychotropic drug effects are mediated by brain neurotransmitters and that some effects, while present, are not significant. They may appear alarming in print, but there is seldom any need to be concerned about them.

### General Effects of Caffeine

Caffeine is classified as a cerebral stimulant. Its administration results in improved psychic and motor performance. There is some question whether this improvement represents an increase over normal levels, or a restoration of normal performance from a state of fatigue. Central nervous system stimulation occurs at all areas, from the cortex to the medulla.

Other parts of the body are affected by caffeine. Heart tissue is directly stimulated; rate and strength of contractions is increased. A cup of coffee may send the blood pressure up five to ten points. The heart's coronary vessels dilate, possibly because of caffeine's direct relaxant effect on smooth muscle. In the stomach, there is increased secretion of hydrochloric acid. In the kidneys, there is reduced reuptake of sodium, with a consequent increase in urine volume, resulting in the familiar copious urination after coffee or tea intake.

The mechanism of action of caffeine, as with most psychotropic drugs, is not clearly established. Current theory holds that there is interference with metabolism of neurotransmitters. The turnover and release of norepinephrine is increased, while turnover of dopamine is decreased. Serotonin levels also rise.

At the molecular level, caffeine increases cellular metabolism by inhibiting an enzyme which degrades a substance that mediates many cellular metabolic processes.

### Absorption, Fate, Excretion, and Dosage

Caffeine may be given orally, rectally, or by injection. It is demethylated and oxidized, and 10 per cent is excreted unchanged. As mentioned above, a cup of brewed coffee contains 100 to 150 mg, which is a therapeutic dose. Instant coffee has about half as much, and decaffeinated coffee about one-fourth.

The 1975 PDR lists twenty-three preparations which contain caffeine. Thirty to 100 mg of caffeine is the usual amount. Up to one gram (1000 mg) may be given by injection.

## Uses

Although caffeine is a component of many preparations, it has few specific uses in psychiatry. It is sometimes employed as a stimulant in elderly or apathetic patients. Some clinicians have tried it with varying success in MBD. One hundred mg of caffeine is about equal to 1 mg of amphetamine in treating MBD. Therefore, the child would need to drink a lot of coffee. There may be other compounds in coffee which affect MBD. Caffeine used to be given I.V. to stimulate the medullary respiratory center in cases of drug overdose. It is seldom used for this purpose currently, as its beneficial effects are equivocal.

## Side Effects

When given in high enough doses to experimental animals, caffeine can cause convulsions, respiratory failure, and death. However, the theoretical fatal dose for man would be 10 gm, so its potential for fatality is low. Caffeine can cause insomnia. It also may cause restlessness, excitement, rapid heart, and even cardiac arrhythmias.

Tolerance to caffeine develops, as some people are capable of drinking large volumes of coffee without excessive stimulation. Recently, attention has been called to the syndrome of *caffeinism*. Symptoms include anxiety, restlessness, headache, insomnia, muscle twitching, and gastrointestinal disturbance. This occurs in individuals who drink eight to fifteen cups of coffee a day. Symptoms disappear when coffee intake is curtailed.

An habitual caffeine user will suffer a minor withdrawal syndrome when intake stops. The main symptoms are headache, restlessness, and fatigue, which usually disappear after a few days.

Identified allergy to caffeine is not reported in the standard literature. Perhaps it has not been looked for.

# SUPPLEMENTARY BIBLIOGRAPHY

## Books

*Advances in Biochemical Psychopharmacology.* New York, Raven, 1974, Vol. 9.

Ayd, Frank (Ed.): *Rational Psychopharmacology and the Right to Treatment.* Baltimore, Ayd Medical Communications, Ltd., 1974.

Barr, Murry L.: *The Human Nervous System - An Anatomical Viewpoint.* New York, Har-Row, 1972.

Benash, Raymond T.: *What is Allergy?* Springfield, Thomas, 1967.

Broch, Samuel and Kruges, Howard P.: *The Basis of Clinical Neurology.* Baltimore, Williams & Wilkins, 1963.

*Dorland's Illustrated Medical Dictionary,* 23rd ed. Philadelphia, Saunders, 1961.

Efran, Daniel H. (Ed.): *Psychopharmacology: A Review of Progress, 1957-1967.* Washington, Public Health Service Publication 1836, 1968.

Elliott, H. Chandler: *Textbook of Neuroanatomy.* Philadelphia, Lippincott, 1963.

Field, John (Ed.): *Handbook of Physiology - Neurophysiology.* Baltimore, Waverly Press, 1960.

Ganay, Wm. T.: *Review of Medical Physiology,* 7th ed. Los Altos, Lange, 1975.

Goodman, Louis, S. and Gilman, Alfred: *The Pharmacological Basis of Therapeutics,* 4th ed. London, Macmillan, 1970.

Goodman, Louis and Gilman, Alfred (Eds.): *The Pharmacological Basis of Therapeutics,* 5th ed. New York, Macmillan, 1975.

Gordon, Maxwell (Ed.): *Psychopharmacological Agents.* New York, Acad Pr, 1967, Vol. II.

Haase, Hans J. and Janssen, Paul A.: *The Action of Neuroleptic Drugs.* Chicago, Year Bk Med, 1965.

Harlow, Harry F. and Woolsey, Clinton N. (Eds.): *Biological & Biochemical Bases of Behavior.* Madison, U of Wis Pr, 1968.

Hollister, Leo E.: *Clinical Use of Psychotherapeutic Drugs.* Springfield, Thomas, 1973.

Humphrey, J. N. and White, R. G.: *Immunology for Students of Medicine.* 3rd Ed., Philadelphia, Davis Co, 1970.

Krupp, Marcus and Chatton, Milton: *Current Diagnosis and Treatment.* Los Altos, Lange, 1972.

Longo, V. G.: *Neuropharmacology and Behavior.* San Francisco, WH Freeman, 1972.

Manter, John T. and Gatz, Arthur J.: *Essentials of Clinical Neuroanatomy & Neurophysiology.* Philadelphia, Davis Co, 1961.

Meyers, Frederick et al.: *Review of Medical Pharmacology.* Los Altos, Lange, 1974.

*Physicians' Desk Reference,* 29th ed. Oradell, Medical Economics, Inc., 1975.

*Scientific Proceedings.* The One Hundred and Twenty-eighth Annual Meeting of the American Psychiatric Association, 1975. American Psychiatric Association, Washington, D.C., April, 1975.

Shepard, Michael et al.: *Clinical Psychopharmacology.* London, English University Press, 1968.

Smith, W. G.: *Allergy and Tissue Metabolism.* London, Wm. Heinemann Medical Books, Ltd., 1964.

Stecker, Paul G. et al.: *The Merck Index,* 8th ed. Rahway, Merck, 1968.

Stevens, Charles F.: *Neurophysiology: A Primer.* New York, Wiley, 1966.

Turk, J. L.: *Immunology in Clinical Medicine.* London, Wm. Heinemann Medical Books, 1967.

Valzelli, Luigi: *Psychopharmacology.* Flushing, Spectrum Publications, Inc., 1973.

Vaughan, Daniel, Cook, Robert, and Asbury, Taylor: *General Ophthalmology,* 3rd ed. Los Altos, Lange, 1962.

Willis, W. D. and Grossman, R. D.: *Medical Neurology.* St. Louis, Mosby, 1973.

## *Journals*

Axelrod, Julius: Neurotransmitters. *Scientific American, 231*:59-71, June, 1974.

Appleton, W. S.: Third psychoactive drug usage guide. *Dis Nerv Syst, 37,1*:39-51, Jan., 1976.

Ayd, F.: A critical evaluation of Molindone (Moban): A new indole derivative neuroleptic. *Dis Nerv Syst, 35,10*:447-452, Oct. 1974.

Ayd, Frank (Ed): Central anticholinergic activity and tricyclic antidepressant efficacy. *Int Drug Ther Newsletter, 10,6*:1-2, June, 1975.

Ayd, Frank; The depot fluphenazines: A reappraisal after ten years' clinical experience. *Am J Psychiatry, 132,5:*491-500, May, 1975.

Bain, J. G., and Turner, T.: Imipramine poisoning. *Arch Dis Child, 46:*887, 1971.

Barron, C. N. et al.: Chlorpromazine and the eye of the dog. *Exp Mol Pathol, 16:*172-179, 1972.

Bidder, George M.: Psychopharmacologic strategies. Lecture, Brentwood V.A. Hospital, January 8, 1976.

Bishop, M. P. and Gallant, D. M.: Loxapine: A controlled evaluation in chronic schizophrenics. *Curr Ther Res, 12,9:*594-597, Sept., 1970.

Blackwell, Barry: Psychotropic drugs in use today. The role of diazepam in medical practice. *JAMA, 225,13:*1637-1641, Sept. 24, 1973.

Breckenridge, R. G.: Cardotoxicity of amitriptyline. *Lancet, 2:*929-930, Oct. 28, 1972.

Cain, R. M. and Cain, Nancy, N.: A compendium of psychoactive drugs, Part I. *Drug Therapy,* 105-124, Jan, 1975.

Carenzi, A. et al.: Dopamine-sensitive adenyl cyclase in human caudate nucleus. *Arch Gen Psychiatry, 32:*1056-1059, Aug., 1975.

Corey, Daniel, and Denny, D.: Deanol in the treatment of tardive dyskinesia. *Am J Psychiatry, 132:*804-807, Aug., 1975.

Coulter, C. et al.: An overdose of parstelin. *Anesthesia, 26,4:*500-501, Oct. 1971.

Crane, George E.: Prevention & management of tardive dyskinesia. *Am J Psychiatry, 129:*466-467, Oct. 1972.

Cunningham, T. A.: Flurazepam hydrochloride - adverse reaction, Clin-Alert, June 13, 1975. (Abstract) *Can Med Assoc J, 112:*805, April 5, 1975.

Cylert: Advertisement in *Psychiatric Annals, 5,5:*80, May, 1975.

Duke, M.: Electrocardiogram of the month: Effects of a psychotropic drug on the electrocardiogram. Imipramine. *Conn Med, 30:*61-63, Jan., 1972.

Drug treatment in psychiatry. Veterans Administration, Washington, D.C., Jan., 1970, Publication.

Eggermont, E. et al.: The adverse influence of imipramine on the adaptation of the newborn infant to extrauterine life. *Acta Paediatr Belg, 26,4:*197-204, 1972.

Everett, H.: The use of bethanecol chloride with tricyclic antidepressants. *Am J Psychiatry, 132,11:*1202-1204, Nov., 1975.

Fejer, D. and Smart, R.: The use of psychoactive drugs by adults. *Can Psychiatric Assoc J, 18,4:*313-319, Aug., 1973.

Fann, W. et al.: Effect of antidepressant and antimanic drugs on amine uptake in man. *J Nerv Ment dis, 158,5:*361-368, 1974.

Fjalland, B. and Nielsen, I.: Methylphenidate antagonism of haloperidol, interaction with cholinergic and anticholinergic drugs. *Psychopharmacologia, 34:*111-118, 1974.

Flemenbaum, A.: Does lithium block the effects of amphetamines? A report of three cases. *Am J Psychiatry, 131,7:*820-821, July, 1974.

Francois, J. and Fener, J.: The effect of phenothiazines on the cell membrane. *Exp Eye Res, 14:*65-68, 1972.

Freeman, J. W. and Coughhead, M. B.: Beta blockade in the treatment of tricyclic antidepressant overdosage. *Med J Aust, 1:*1233-1235, 1973.

Friedenberg, W. et al.: Intravenous diazepam administration. *JAMA, 224,6:*901, May 7, 1973.

Gershon, Samuel: Lithium. *Rational Drug Therapy, 5,7:*1-5, July, 1971.

Granacher, R. P. and Baldessarini, R. J.: Physostigmine - its use in acute anticholinergic syndrome with antidepressant and antiparkinsonian drugs. *Arch Gen Psychiatry, 32:*375-380, March, 1975.

Graves, James E.: The long-acting phenothiazines. *Arch Gen Psychiatry, 32:*893-900, July, 1975.

Greden, John F.: Anxiety or caffeinism: A diagnostic dilemma. *Am J Psychiatry, 131,10:*1089-1092, Oct., 1974.

Greenblatt, D. and Shader, R. I.: Rational use of psychotropic drugs II. antianxiety agents. *J Maine Med Assoc, 64,9:*225-229, Sept., 1974.

Hackett, Thomas P. and Cassem, N. H.: Reduction of anxiety in the coronary care unit. A controlled double-blind comparison of chlordiazepoxide and amobarbital. *Curr Ther Res, 14,10:*649-656, Oct., 1972.

Himwich, H. and Alpers, H.: Psychopharmacology. *Ann Rev of Pharmacology,* 313-333, 1970.

Hollister, Leo: New developments in psychotherapeutic drugs. *Psychiatry Digest, 36,3:*11-22, March, 1975.

Ishak, K. G., and Irey, N.: Hepatic injury associated with the phenothiazines. *Arch Pathol, 93:*283-304, April, 1972.

Janowsky, D. et al.: Antagonistic effects of physostigmine and methylphenidate in man. *Am J Psychiatry, 130,12:*1370-1376, Dec., 1973.

Johnson, Walter C.: A neglected modality in psychiatric treatment - the monoamine oxidase inhibitors. *Dis Nerv Syst, 36,9:*521-525, Sept. 1975.

Kantor, S. J. et al.: Imipramine-induced heart block. *JAMA, 231,13:*1364-1366, March 31, 1975.

Kiev, Ari: The chemotherapy of depressive illness. *Drug Therapy, 1,* 2:9-14, Feb., 1971.

Klawans, Harold L. et al.: A pharmacological model of the pathophysiology of schizophrenia. *Dis Nerv Syst*, 267-275, May, 1975.

Langdon, D. E. et al.: Thrombophlebitis with diazepam used intravenously. *JAMA, 232,2:*184-185, Jan. 8, 1973.

Lipman, A. G.: Drug interactions involving antidepressant agents. *Mod Med, 43:*79-80, Sept. 1, 1975.

Lipman, A. G.: Drug interactions involving antidepressant agents. *Mod Med, 43,17:*69, Oct. 1, 1975.

Litvak, R. and Kaeling, R.: Dermatological side effects with psychotropics. *Dis Nerv Syst*, 309-311, May, 1972.

Lutz, E. G.: Allergic conjunctivitis due to diazepam. *Am J Psychiatry, 132,5:*548, May, 1975.

Manber, M.: The medical effects of coffee. *Medical World News, 17,2:*63-73, Jan. 26, 1976.

Mandell, A. J.: Neurological barriers to euphoria. *Am Sci, 61:*565-573, Sept.-Oct., 1973.

Matsuki, A. et al.: Excessive mortality in schizophrenic patients on chronic phenothiazine treatment. *Aggressologie, 13:*407-418, 1972.

Moban: Endo Laboratories, Garden City, New York, Advertisement Pamphlet.

Moir, D. C. et al.: Cardiotoxicity of amitriptyline. *Lancet, 2:*561-564, Sept. 16, 1972.

Neurological syndromes associated with antipsychotic drug use. Editorial in *Arch Gen Psychiatry, 28:*463-467, April, 1973.

North, Richard R.: Drug induced movement. *Postgrad Med, 50:*180-185, Sept. 1971.

Parker, J. D. and Fenton, G. W.: Levo (-) amphetamine and dextro (+) amphetamine in the treatment of narcolepsy. *J Neurol, Neurosurg & Psychiatry, 36:*1076-1081, 1973.

Petti, T. and Campbell, M.: Imipramine & seizures. *Am J Psychiatry, 132,5:*538-540, May, 1975.

Possaint, Alvin F. and Ditman, Keith S.: A controlled study of imipramine (Tofranil) in the treatment of childhood enuresis. *J Pediatr, 67,2:*283-290, Aug., 1965.

Side effects of psychotropic drugs. *Psychiatric Annals, 5:*entire issue. Nov., 1972.

Raskin, David E.: Akathisia: A side effect to be remembered. *Am J Psychiatry, 129,3:*345-347, Sept., 1972.

Reda, F. A. et al.: Lithium carbonate in the treatment of tardive dyskinesia. *Am J Psychiatry, 132,5:*560-562, May, 1975.

Schnackenberg, R. C.: Caffeine as a substitute for Schedule II stimulants in hyperkinetic children. *Am J Psychiatry, 130:*796-

798, 1973.

Sessa, Anna et al.: Propranalol in imipramine poisoning. *Am J Dis Child, 126:*847-849, Dec., 1973.

Shapiro, Arthur K.: Rational use of psychopharmaceutic agents. *N Y State of J Med, 64,9:*1084-1095, May 1, 1964.

Shapsin, B. and Gershon, S.: Cogwheel rigidity related to lithium maintenance. *Am J Psychiatry, 132,5:*536-538, May, 1975.

Simpson, G. M. et al.: Clinical pharmacological trial of loxapine succinate. *J Clin Pharmacol, 10,3:*175-181, May-June, 1970.

Siomopoulos, V.: Amphetamine psychosis: Overview and a hypothesis. *Dis Nerv Syst, 36,6:*336-338, June, 1975.

Small, J. G. et al.: A placebo-controlled study of lithium carbonate combined with neuroleptics in chronic schizophrenic patients. *Am J Psychiatry, 132,12:*1315-1317, December, 1975.

Snyder, S. et al.: Antischizophrenic drugs and brain cholinergic receptors. *Arch Gen Psychiatry, 31:*58-61, July, 1974.

Snyder, Solomon N. et al.: Drugs, neurotransmitters, and schizophrenia. *Science, 184:*1243-1253, June 21, 1974.

Stowartz, R. J. et al.: On the significance of the increase in homovanillic acid (HVA) caused by antipsychotic drugs in corpus striatum and limbic forebrain. *Psychopharmacologia, 43, 2:* 1975.

Thearle, M. B. and Dunn, P. M.: Exchange transfusion for diazepam intoxication at birth followed by jejunal stenosis. *Proc R Soc Med, 66:*349-350, April, 1973.

Tranquilizers causing aggression. Editorial in *Br Med J, 149:*113-114, Jan. 18, 1975.

Van Eyk, R. and Bots, G.: Psychopharmacological agents and cerebral oedema. *Psychiatr Neurol Neurochir (Amsterdam), 75:*61-67, 1972.

Young, Anne B. et al.: Interaction of benzodiazepines with central nervous glycine receptors: Possible mechanism of action. *Proc Natl Acad Sci USA, 71,6:*2246-2250, June, 1974.

# INDEX

163